BLOOD IN MY COFFEE

THE LIFE OF THE FIGHT DOCTOR

FERDIE PACHECO

SPORTS
PUBLISHING

Sports Publishing books may be purchased in bulk at special discounts for sales promotion, corporate gifts, fund-raising, or educational purposes. Special editions can also be created to specifications. For details, contact the Special Sales Department, Sports Publishing, 307 West 36th Street, 11th Floor, New York, NY 10018 or sportspub-books@skyhorsepublishing.com.

Sports Publishing® is a registered trademark of Skyhorse Publishing, Inc.®, a Delaware corporation.

Visit our website at www.sportspubbooks.com.

10 9 8 7 6 5 4 3 2 1

Library of Congress Cataloging-in-Publication Data is available on file.

ISBN: 978-1-61321-197-7

Printed in China

This book is primarily dedicated to my wife, Luisita a.k.a. Karen Maestas, my partner until death do us part, helping and guiding me through the hard places in life, and enjoying the victories together. Thirty-four years of bliss have passed, living in peace and tranquility in Miami. Luisita has typed and edited all 15 of my books. She is a source of inspiration. She is my reason for living. If you have any criticisms of this book, e-mail Luisita. It's as much her book as it is mine.

And to our daughter, Tina, who traveled with us on many boxing journeys and helped with the edit of this book.

A special dedication to a courageous man, Mills Lane. A Marine Corps combat veteran, a famous law man, a high-court judge, and the best boxing referee in the history of the sport. He is currently fighting a courageous battle to recover from a stroke, and our prayers are with him.

OTHER BOOKS BY FERDIE PACHECO

Non-Fiction
Fight Doctor
Muhammad Ali: A View from the Corner
Ybor City Chronicles
Columbia Restaurant Cook Book
Pacheco's Art of Ybor City
Christmas Eve Cookbook
Pacheco's Art of Cubans in Exile
The 12 Greatest Rounds of Boxing
Nino Peretti's Caffe Abbracci Cookbook
Tales of the 5th Street Gym

Fiction
Renegade Lightning
Who Killed Patton?
(for young readers)
Trolley Kat Travels
Trolley Kat ABC

ferdiepacheco.com

CONTENTS

FOREWORD

I've met a lot of people in my life from Charles Lindbergh and Charlie Chaplin to Scott Fitzgerald and John Steinbeck to Marlon Brando, and Muhammad Ali. If I had to pick the single-most unequal, I would have to nominate Dr. Ferdie Pacheco.

People count themselves blessed when they're gifted with a talent. So what do you say to Pacheco, the ghetto doctor who became a corner man for Muhammad Ali, who wrote excellent books on boxing, and who became a boxing announcer—that's only the beginning. A distinguished painter, he's also a novelist and a war historian, and what I find most appealing about Ferdie is his tireless creative enthusiasm.

—Budd Schulberg

ACKNOWLEDGMENTS

When a man who has had multiple successful careers writes a book when he is in the golden years, the list of acknowledgments should read like a phone book. I will try to list the many people who read, commented, gave advice, and were of great assistance in this book. Forgive me if I forget a few. It's the price of old age. Just know that I do feel grateful for all the help given to me.

Most book acknowledgments begin with the first step taken, and that is approval from the wife. My wife, Luisita, was the prime encouragement to begin the autobiography, and then served as my typist and the initial editor of the first rough draft. Her work was indispensable to the book.

Thank you goes to everyone here: to the fellow writers who got the first copies of my autobiography, Budd Schulberg, novelist and screenwriter; Richard Prachter, *Miami Herald* writer; and Pat Keen, military historian, who helped with the edit. Carl Hiaasen, novelist and columnist for the *Miami Herald*; Dave Barry, novelist and columnist for the *Miami Herald*; Ed Pope, sports editor of the *Miami Herald*; Howard Kleinberg of the *Miami News*; David Lawrence, publisher of the *Miami Herald*; Edna Buchanan, mystery writer; Les Standiford; mystery writer and director of creative writing at FIU, Dan Wakefield; novelist and professor, Pauline Winick; Kevin Monaghan, NBC executive; John Gonzales, NBC director; NBC producer Mike Weisman; and Thomas Hauser (whose remark was "Who the f--- wants to read a biography of you?"). Bob Skimin, military historian and novelist; *Sports Illustrated*'s Pat Putnam; *Tampa Tribune* editorial writer Joe Guidry; Pat Manteiga of the *La Gaceta* newspaper; Mitch Kaplan of Books and Books; Jack Heaney former UPI writer; Lou Duva and Kathy Duva; and Sally Richardson of St. Martin's Press, who introduced me to my literary agent, Tony Seidl, who introduced me to Bob Snodgrass, my present agent. Finally, Professor Gary Mormino, USF history department for encouraging me to write about Ybor City history.

Thankfully they were all encouraging, critical, and complimentary. I cut some stuff (there are libel laws), added a tiny bit, but 95 percent of the book stood the test of their scrutiny, and I pushed forward.

When the book was first compiled it came to 700 pages. The expertise furnished to chop this down to 238 pages came from an amazing editor, Matt Fulks. Working with him was an incredibly pleasurable experience. We sat down one weekend at my home in Miami, and by Monday had the finished book. Now, that is editing!

CHAPTER 1

Death Is Never Far

I was happy to be seated at ringside as the analyst for the Sugar Ray Leonard versus Roberto Duran fight in Montreal on a hot night. It was a pay-per-view fight, so instead of working for NBC—my network at the time—promoter Bob Arum hired me. He appointed Bill Mazur, a baseball broadcaster, to be my blow-by-blow partner.

I loved Mazur, because he was an old-time New York guy from the 1940s and 1950s, whose shtick on his radio show was his phenomenal memory of baseball trivia. And best of all, he had a red wig that had turned orange.

The last thing on my mind on June 20, 1980, was death, my old companion in my medical office of the ghetto in Miami. Death is never far away there. I came to find out that death is never far away in the ring either.

The main undercard fight was a revenge-bout between Canadian Gaeton Hart and American Cleveland Denny. They were two top-ranked fighters who hated each other. If there was a moment's pause, it was that Cleveland Denny had taken some big beatings in his previous few bouts.

For five rounds in Montreal, they hammered away at each other. An even fight. Then the fight swung dramatically to Gaeton Hart's favor: Denny faded, he tired, and he was losing each round decisively. I started to criticize the referee for not stopping the fight. Death had stepped into the arena.

A few rounds later, Hart caught Denny in the corner. Denny was defenseless. Hart started a two-handed barrage of hard punches. The

Canadian crowd, on its feet, roared. The media people at ringside were also on their feet, but screaming for the referee to stop the fight. He didn't. Cleveland slumped to the canvas. Hart stood over him, arms upraised in triumph, ready for Cleveland to get up, but he never did.

I saw Denny's handlers try to pry the mouthpiece out of his mouth. They couldn't. His mouth was shut so tight that a crowbar couldn't open his jaws. Where was the doctor? Nowhere in sight (turns out he was in the upper deck trying to buy a hot dog)! Where were the paramedics? There were none. Where was the ambulance? There was no ambulance?

I knew then that essentially Cleveland Denny was a dead man.

When the brain explodes and a cascade of blood courses down between the two hemispheres of the brain, it short-circuits all of the wires. The nerve trunks, which affect the spasms of the jaw muscle, are cut, and there is nothing to keep it from clapping shut. Nothing can unclamp it.

An impulse to help the poor man came over me. I ripped off my headphones and rushed into the ring to help until they found the doctor and ordered an ambulance. Mazur looked at me as is if I'd lost my mind. He was from the world of journalism, trained to observe and report. Mine was a medical training: I observed, diagnosed, and did something about it.

Of course, I knew I could not save Denny. I held him in my arms until he died. I put him in the ambulance that would rush him to surgery to operate. But the doctors were operating on a corpse.

✗✗✗✗✗✗

I left Canada resolved to make sure that there would not be another NBC telecast unless the promoter signed a contract to provide an ambulance with paramedics and that the boxing commission would see to it that there was always a doctor at ringside.

When I got back to New York, I went straight to NBC executive producer Don Ohlmeyer, told him of the horrifying night, and asked permission to use NBC to attack boxing's cavalier attitude toward death in the ring.

Ideally, no boxing would take place on NBC shows without a contract for an ambulance in place at ringside. No ambulance, no fight. I can't tell you how gutsy a call that was for Ohlmeyer and NBC president Arthur Watson. Eventually we won. Today there are ambulances at all bouts because of NBC.

After a bit of shouting, ABC and CBS followed suit, and now HBO and Showtime have that clause in their contracts. I have to credit Ohlmeyer, who broke the mold of "We only televise it, we're not part of it," and didn't stand in my way. He just said, "Do it," and I did.

Throughout my years of freedom in front of an NBC microphone, I campaigned mightily to change things in boxing. Some battles I won, some I lost, but I still tried. We led the fight and changed a great many faults, which in turn diminished boxing deaths.

I fought for the installation of a fourth rope on the boxing ring to keep heads from bouncing on the ring apron. A four-rope ring is now standard. I also fought for a different glove design, one where the thumb would be attached to the glove. As it was, the thumb was a missile that could take out an eye. That idea passed throughout the world. The hardest fight of all, though, was the one major improvement I talked about in the beginning—having an ambulance and a doctor at every fight. I am proud it is now standard practice.

One of the biggest battles was the change in the attitude of referees and cornermen when it came to stopping a fight. Historically, the promoter and the crowd wanted to see a match to the finish. Stopping a fight prematurely was considered the end of the career. No one wanted a merciful referee. Merciful officials never worked another fight!

I came blasting into the picture with a microphone and direct scathing criticism of insanely bolder referees. No longer would we refuse to identify them by name. Now, every guilty referee, cornerman, or manager was called by name. Slow-motion replays magnified mistakes. With clever evidence of mistakes and of the reluctance to stop the beating, and with their names clearly on national television, they started to change.

Before a fight, at the weigh-in, and halls, they would sidle up to me.

"Please don't call my name," they pleaded. "My family is catching hell because of what you're saying about me."

"Well my boy, just do your job. Don't fuck up. Don't cause a death, and you'll not hear your name, except in praise when you do your job right," I'd say.

Slowly, boxing became more humane. For that permission to attack the guilty ruthlessly, I give my public thanks to Don Ohlmeyer and the late Arthur Watson. We had many small victories with the commissions, boxing managers, trainers, and referees. I was proud of the work we did and the record we left.

Only Fighters Die

Of the many things I saw in the boxing ring that I could not condone, nor find an excuse for, nor fit into my code of life, was the death of a boxer. Every time I was a witness to, or part of a boxing death, I came home to sleepless nights. Why was I, an ethical physician, with a large charity practice, a part of a sport that allowed death to be a part of the sport? Why was I part of the corner work, which encouraged, exhorted, and sent one man to hurt the other to the point where death results? I never found a suitable answer. I don't have one now. I don't know if there is one. I suppose I have to say it's a character flaw.

I believe the main reason for death, though, is a big beating the fighter sustains in a previous bout. This is entirely avoidable. Good record keeping, computerized records, instantly available, and a boxing commission with balls would prevent those deaths. In the avoidable Emile Griffith versus Benny "Kid" Paret, a cursory review of Paret's record would have revealed that Paret took a monstrous beating at the hands of Gene Fullmer, a middleweight with a heavy punch. Paret's brain was softened up. It blew up on him against Griffith.

My first death in the ring occurred in 1963, when Ultiminio "Sugar" Ramos ended the life of the "Springfield Rifle," Davey Moore. Those were the days of three-strand ropes. Had there been four strands, Davey's head would have stopped instead of slamming onto the hard canvas floor.

✗✗✗✗✗✗✗

By pushing for safety issues in boxing, I put a huge band-aid on my conscience for the sins I had committed when I worked in the corners. I think there are fewer deaths now and fewer fearful beatings. In addition, regrettably, there are fewer loud-mouthed announcers willing to identify and criticize incompetent officials and bad rules. And, as with everything in boxing, old habits slide back in. Money talks. Old washed-up fighters keep fighting, plodding on doggedly, defeat after defeat, into neurological damage, or the punch-drunk syndrome, Parkinson's disease or Alzheimer's, and, eventually, death. Why? Because the "public wants to see it," which translates to money and ratings. As one of the old gray men of Miami's famed Fifth Street Gym said to me: *"Only the fighters die."*

CHAPTER 2

Following My Hero

You could call me almost famous.

Almost famous? Sure, it's a curious phenomenon usually associated with second bananas. Jackie Gleason was famous. Art Carney was almost famous. Movie stars are famous; character actors are almost famous. George Clooney is famous. Steve Buscemi is—well, you get the idea. In boxing, Muhammad Ali was (and is) a superstar. His trainer, Angelo Dundee, was almost famous. Me, too. I was Ali's personal physician for 17 years. I've also been a boxing analyst (among other things), but I've never been famous.

It's nice to be known but still move unimpeded through the day. I get a good table at restaurants, tickets to sold-out Broadway shows, hotel rooms, and seats on overbooked flights, and very few hassles and obligations in exchange for these courtesies. Who could complain about that? Not me. I'm almost famous.

Fortunately, my lack of universal recognition (the *almost* part) doesn't let me get too spoiled. Once, at a boxing match in Miami, I found myself surrounded by autograph seekers and couldn't see the ring. I noticed an empty seat next to *Miami Herald* sports editor Edwin Pope and his wife. Pope got up and went to the dressing room to interview a fighter. I took a chance, leaped into the empty seat, turned my back to the passing fans, and got into a deep conversation with Mrs. Pope.

The guys sitting behind us immediately nailed me for an autograph. Then I felt a presence in front of me. I didn't look up and hoped that whoever stood there would take the hint and leave. He did not. It was Christmastime, so I kind of waved and mumbled, "Merry Christmas" in his direction.

"Merry Christmas," he responded but still didn't budge.

I stared up at him. He had nothing in his hand; no pen, no paper. I got mad.

"You got a piece of paper?" I asked.

"No, I haven't," he said.

One of the guys behind me took pity, tore off a piece of his program, and handed it to me.

"I don't suppose you have a pen?" I asked, dripping sarcasm.

"No, I haven't," he replied.

Another guy behind me produced a pen.

I grabbed it, scribbled my autograph, and handed it to the impassive gent.

"Listen, Bub. Any time you ask someone for an autograph, make sure you at least have a paper and pencil," I muttered.

I was hot.

Squinting at my autograph as if it was a hieroglyphic, he said, sweetly, "I don't know who you are, sir, but you're in my seat. I'd just like to sit down."

I've had a few of those moments in my 25 years of being almost famous. Hubris, it's called, and it reminds me who I really am and from where I came.

Papa's Influence

I was born in Ybor City, the Spanish quarter of Tampa, Florida, on December 8, 1927, in the home of my grandfather, Gustavo Jimenez. My father, J.B. Pacheco, was a pharmacist. As was customary, he and his wife, Consuelo (my mother), lived with my mother's parents until they saved enough to purchase their own home.

J.B. and Gustavo—two powerful and unusual men—deeply influenced me. They showed me how to get the most out of what God had given me, to love learning, to live a decent life, and in time, how to become as worldly and honorable as them—and to make a difference in the world.

My father, the monolithic heroic figure, worked seven days a week from 8 a.m. until 11 p.m. at his pharmacy, La Economica. With whatever free time he had, he played cards and dabbled in politics in the cellar of the Centro Asturiano Club, the social center of our community.

So, my grandfather served as male authority figure and mentor to my older brother, Joseph, and me. My grandfather had botched the job badly with his own seven children, and he knew it. Hard discipline hadn't worked in the New World, so when we came along, he regarded us as his second chance and spent all of his spare time educating us in a gentle and loving manner.

Because Gustavo Jimenez had been a concert flautist, he wanted to cultivate our creative sides. Both my brother and I demonstrated a flair for art but had no talent for music. Regardless, we were forced to listen to the Metropolitan Opera Company on the radio in his study every Saturday, as announcer Milton Cross gave a blow-by-blow description of the action (or lack of it). Consequently, I have hated opera all my life.

Sunday was somewhat better. Grandfather would hand me a No. 2 pencil, pick me up, and put me on a chair, and I conducted the NBC Symphony Orchestra along with Maestro Arturo Toscanini. I'd wave the pencil back and forth in front of the radio, pretending to be a conductor. I learned about the tempo and rhythms of classical music and knew most major symphonies before I was nine. I loved them all, particularly Beethoven, Mozart, and especially Rachmaninoff and Tchaikovsky.

My grandfather decided that we should get to know the paintings of the Renaissance masters, which hung in nearby Sarasota at the Ringling Museum of Art (affiliated with and supported by the Ringling Bros. Circus). It was great, but if Grandfather thought that those masterworks would inspire us to become painters, they elicited the opposite effect on Joseph and me. We wondered how in the hell we were ever supposed to paint like that.

It wasn't until much later, after discovering the apparent simplicity of impressionists such as Van Gogh, Lautrec, Monet, and the rest, I thought, "Hell, I can do that!"

Taking the long way home from Sarasota on our trips, we stopped at the beautiful botanical gardens of Bok Towers in Lake Worth. We'd spread our blanket; pull out a big thermos of dark, rich, and thick Spanish cocoa; and tear open boxes of Social Tea crackers, which we covered with butter and jam. We sat quietly, listening to the lovely music of the chimes while my grandfather patiently explained the benefits of meditation. This was years before rock stars and movie starlets traveled to India and meditation became popular in the West.

Therefore, you see, from early on, I was quite cool. I just didn't know it. (However, it was hard to figure out on what to meditate when I was six years of age!)

The most meaningful and lasting of Grandfather's contributions to our education also came on Sundays. My grandmother, Carmen, joined the three of us. We rode the 3 p.m. streetcar downtown for our weekly treat, a first-run MGM movie, at the fabulous Tampa Theater. Its Renaissance architecture, in the style of a Venetian Doge's palace, was magnificent. Fascinated by the dialogue and actions of the beautiful people on the screen, I clutched Grandfather's hand, trying to grasp the intricacies of the plot.

After the movie, we boarded the streetcar and returned home. My grandmother broke out the hot chocolate and churros (little stuffed and fried pastries). Then, the fun began. My grandfather, speaking in a professorial manner, lectured and explained the plot of the movie to us. He'd finish his summation, and it all made sense. After all, Joseph and I were young geniuses (or so we were told), and movies weren't very deep.

"But that's not the way it was at all," my grandmother said.

She had come to America when she was 19 and never spoke a word of English, so her interpretations of the movies diverged wildly from the plot. They triggered many healthy arguments between my grandparents that were almost as entertaining as the original movies.

As a musician, Grandfather loved Fred Astaire and Ginger Rogers movies. He made us watch those films three times! A first viewing was just to watch Fred Astaire. He was a genius when he danced, so we concentrated on him alone. The second viewing was a study of Ginger Rogers.

"She is almost as good as Mr. Astaire, but remember she dances backward while wearing high heels and a very heavy dress!" Grandfather would remind us.

We also loved the musical production numbers and the performances of the great comic character actors such as Eric Blore and Edward Everett Horton.

The third viewing, we just relaxed and took in the whole film—flimsy plot and all.

As you see, life in our wonderful family home was like being in a university. There were always books to read, movies to see, radio programs to hear—and everything to examine and discuss. Our hungry young minds soaked it all up, and we were never bored.

My brother and I learned about the world outside Ybor City as no other kids in town did. Our family home was also the Tampa headquarters for the Loyalists during the Spanish Civil War, which had started in 1936 when I was nine years old. Our parlor was filled with refugees, veterans, wounded soldiers, and other human detritus from that war.

Once, we cared for a captain from the International Brigades who was shot through both cheeks. One side of his face had healed, but not the other, which he left open, he said, for recruiting purposes, although how seeing this awful injury could inspire a kid to fight, I would never guess. Eating supper with him at our family table was an experience not easily forgotten.

My grandfather and I kept military situation maps to track the war news. Every morning, when the communiqués came in, we stuck red pins in the map. I loved it when my grandfather, in his serious, authoritative voice said, "All quiet on the western front," echoing the title of the movie by that name we saw downtown.

By 1938, the Loyalists were defeated, and so was my grandfather. He died, it seems to me, just as the Fascists triumphed.

Grandma gave each of us a dime and sent us to the corner ice cream store for a double-dip cone. Nevertheless, it was a sad time for us. To this day, I miss Grandfather's soft, educated voice, his aristocratic demeanor, and his warm hugs.

✗✗✗✗✗✗

My father then took over our education. He had apparently waited until we were old enough to be taught about his world, which had nothing at all to do with art or music or drama. His world was science and healing.

My father's family boasted generations of pharmacists and doctors—going back several centuries. He was totally committed to the idea that God had delivered two geniuses into his big hands, and His message was clear: They would become physicians and help the poor.

My brother, Joseph, was too delicate for blood and gore. Although he had undeniable brainpower, he rebelled in his own way with a series of nervous breakdowns until he got wise, left town, and moved as far away from my father as he could, to California. He taught English at the University of San Francisco.

So I became the focus of my father's considerable attention and welcomed it. Papa was Hercules, Aristotle, and Franklin D. Roosevelt rolled into one tough, broad-backed, ham-fisted Superman.

Once a guy tried to steal our parking place just as we began backing into it. Papa quickly hit the brakes, got out, pulled the man halfway out his car's window, popped him with a straight right, and regained his rightful parking space while I looked on in wide-eyed amazement.

One of the many ways he showed his affection for me was the bizarre things he did to objects that "attacked" me.

My grandmother had an old black iron fork she used for heavy cooking (don't ask). It had been in her family for centuries. Once, I stepped on it and punctured my foot. My father rushed home, administered a tetanus shot, patched it up, and then snarled, "Show me the fork that did this to you."

He glared at the offending fork, grabbed it, opened the back door, and flung it as far as he could. We never saw it again. This made Grandma sore as hell and she never forgave my father, who could not have cared less.

But Papa was easy to talk to, and I could always make him laugh. Every morning, I sat on the side of the bathtub and watched him as he shaved and dressed for work. It was our time together. One time, I saw him put his shirt and trousers on, grab a huge .45 automatic pistol, and stick it in his belt, just before he put on his coat.

Boy was that cool! How many kids had a dad who carried a .45 pistol—and also slept with it under his pillow? It was years before I asked myself, "Wait a minute, since when does a pharmacist carry a .45?"

Once, about 2 a.m., I had to go to the bathroom. I was too sleepy to turn the light on. I groggily padded through the house, and the next thing I knew, I faced the business end of his .45. I briefly considered reverting to bed-wetting, but boy, it was oh so cool to know my dad guarded our house. Nazi spies, burglars, and such did not stand a chance!

✗✗✗✗✗✗

With World War II looming on the horizon, Papa came home with the news that he had bought La Economica Drugstore on 16th Street and Columbus Drive, across from the Regensburg Cigar Factory, or El Reloj as we knew it.

It never occurred to me to ask what my father did for a living. Because of Sweet Sam, our deliveryman, I knew Papa was the head of Sharpe and Dome Pharmaceuticals. However, with my brother and me growing up, our future held the cost of medical school, and my father, a smart businessman, considered that he would need a business to pillage and defray the costs of our education. We bought La Economica from Dr. Rubio who lived next door.

During this time, as my father was building up the store, I was working as a waiter at the Columbia Café Shop. Some weeks I'd make $50 and even $60 a week in tips. My father did not let Lawrence, the owner, pay me a waiter's salary $28 a week. I got $6 a week because I was 14 and, therefore, was not entitled to a man's salary. I spread that story around, and my tips tripled! I loved to work there. Air-conditioned, three free meals a day, and tips. To my considerable astonishment, one day my father brought me to the store and announced that my Columbia Café days were over. From now on, I would apprentice in pharmacy under him, as he had under his dad.

Now, I was thunderstruck. I was sad as hell to do without the Columbia fun and pizzazz, the air-conditioning (a very big plus in the hot Tampa summer), and three delicious Columbia meals a day. In exchange, I found myself in a tiny box-like drugstore, without any air-conditioning or ventilation that was a dust bowl from the incoming air of the street. No soda fountain. My father was an ethical pharmacist and hated soda fountains. We were, what the English call, *chemists*.

The other outstanding negative aspect of my change of profession from waiter to chemist was roughly $50. I found my father did not intend to pay me. At all. Zippo. Zero. Of course, I could ask for money that I needed (the operative word is *ask*). He never turned me down. I asked for money to go to a movie theater, though, and he gave me the bare bones, a dime—the price of admission for a child. No carfare, no candy, no popcorn, no Coca-Cola. Then I sprung up and grew taller, and the cashier gave me the fisheye with my dime for admission. When I told my dad, he said, "Crouch down." I never knew if he was kidding.

It's then that I formulated a "don't make waves" attitude. He gave me a dime, and I took a quarter from the cash register. I was never sure whether he knew, but somehow it worked out. Hell, I was 17 years old, and he still was giving me a dime.

I think the dime thing might have run in the family. Uncle Ralph, a double amputee, came to do our books every month. I would rush out to see him (I was always glad to see a relative) and help him carry his books. Invariably Ralph gave me a dime. Invariably, and inevitably, he never changed. After I graduated and became a registered pharmacist, I took over the drugstore as its proprietor. Still, when my uncle brought his legless self in to do the books on the prescription counter, he only gave me a dime.

My father's explanation to me was that if I helped him run the drugstore now, during the war when there were no men available, he would in turn send me to college and medical school at a first-class university. This made sense to me, and because I worshipped my father, I was bursting with pride that I was needed to help the family. It never occurred to me that sending me to college was my father's obligation. He was supposed to do that. I never questioned it. To this day I don't. He lived to send me to four years of premed and died before he could help pay for my medical school. The sale of La Economica Drugstore helped me pay my way through medical school. So in a way, I guess it all worked out.

For my part, I never regretted one hour in that oven of a drugstore. The main thing was I was working next to my father, learning his profession. My idolization of my father grew and grew in my estimation. He was a tower of strength. He was very correct and very moral, and he was super-intelligent, the brightest guy I knew except possibly for the lector Victoriano Manteiga. To me, my father was a giant, and I luxuriated in his shadow; I felt warmed and protected by his approving eye. He never laid a hand on me, perhaps because of his father's brutality, and rarely scolded me. He was very patient with my foibles and craziness as a practical joker and seemed to get pleasure from hearing of my wild escapades. I never did anything illegal or wrong, because I couldn't stand to disappoint him. I'd rather take a whipping than hurt or disappoint my father.

It took me years to work all this out, because Papa was an enigma. That made him all the more interesting. It wasn't until I started writing *The Ybor City Chronicles* that I found out about my father's mafia connections. He was known as "The Philosopher," because his job was to mediate squabbles within the mafia and the police, politicians, or rival gangs to avoid gunplay and keep things peaceful. His word was law. He was very intelligent and had a lot of common sense. No wonder he slept with a .45 automatic under his pillow and always carried it in his back belt. Of whom was he wary? I never knew. He never volunteered, I sure didn't ask. I knew that once he and Lawrence had survived an assassination attempt, but they never talked about it.

Another thing I recently found out was that all during that terrible depression of the 1930s, we had money! Boy, you could have fooled me! My father acted poor. I got a dime for lunch from elementary school through high school. A dime! A hot dog and chocolate milk. He never took us to school or came to pick us up after school, even if it was raining cats and dogs. We walked home. Not even a nickel for the streetcar.

Why? Well, that money fell under the responsibility of my mother. That was *house* money. School matters were her responsibility. My father was off in the drug store world from 8:00 a.m. to 11:00 p.m.

Papa always dressed in a blue serge suit. His clothes fit well. He wore hats all the time and two-toned shoes. He always smelled great. I loved to hug him because of the smell of his aftershave lotion. And of course the thrill of seeing him put the Colt automatic in his back pocket. He was some cool dude!

At La Economica Drugstore, we always had a registered pharmacist splitting a shift with him. The pharmacists were a varied lot. We went through several losers until we lucked out on a super pharmacist and an exemplary human being. Dr. Gus Moreno II was a widower with a son of my age, Gus III, who went to Spring Hill College with me and eventually was my roommate. He went on to be an obstetrician. We were a tight, happy family. Initially after my father died suddenly, Gus bought the drugstore, which helped me pay for medical school.

One experience I remember vividly was a disastrous trial employment of a very proud, very stiff Spaniard who somehow acquired a license despite the fact that he couldn't speak English.

He would station himself behind the counter, acting as if he were reading the *Tampa Tribune*. The fact that he spoke no English infuriated Papa. In addition he did no manufacturing and packaging. The final straw came when my father, while in the back making five gallons of elixir of terpin hydrate and codeine, overheard the following conversation.

"I have a feverish achy feeling all over my body, runny nose, sore throat, and a cough which won't go away," a female customer explained. "What shall I get?"

"Fix a big cup of manzanilla tea, put two lemons, and a tablespoon of honey, and get in bed for two days," Dr. Rivero responded.

"That's all?"

"If you're not well in two days, stay in bed for two more days."

"That's all?"

"If you're not well by then, come back and I'll give you medicine for the flu. Then get back in bed for two days."

She left, rather disappointed and shocked. My father, who had a mere mercurial temper, came storming out of the back.

"Listen here, Rivero, we are not selling furniture in here. We don't sell beds. What we sell is medicine! Medicine to cure the flu!"

And with that Papa tossed out Dr. Rivero. I was glad to see the pompous little guy leave. For one thing, it killed me when he would hold the *Tampa Tribune* out at arms length and read the headlines. "Chin Chin Howzer says landing soon!" To hear Eisenhower's name so mangled made me boil.

✗✗✗✗✗✗

My father really taught me about every aspect of life. He had rules of conduct—principles—and would not deviate from them if he felt he was right. That ultimately got me into a lot of trouble with NBC, Showtime, the military, and various hospitals, but I still abide by what he taught me. As a result, I've lived a scrupulously decent life and have never had a bad night's sleep from an aching conscience. Here is a partial list of his rules:

1. Always be yourself. Don't try to be like anyone else. You are you. Let others try to be like you.

2. Never lie if you can help it. Little lies don't count. You can tell a sick person he looks good, or an ugly girl she looks pretty. Don't lie about important things. It's too hard to remember lies. Tell the truth and stick to your guns, lies come back to bite you on the ass.

3. Pick the best girl you can find and marry her for life. Stay faithful, it's the easiest way.

4. Never take a partner; if you succeed, he takes half the credit. If you fail, you take all the blame. Live or die in business on your own two feet. You take all the credit and all the blame.

5. Never do a good deed and brag about it. Otherwise, you haven't done a damn thing but something for yourself.

6. Never brag, never call attention to what you do well. If you've a brain or can paint or play the piano, God is to be given credit, not you.

7. Don't ask for money as a loan. Go hungry first. Don't loan money, either. You lose the money and the friend.

8. Don't tell secrets. A secret can be kept only when you tell one person—yourself.

9. Never bet on a game that is played with a ball that is not round.

10. When you shake someone's hand look him or her straight in the eyes and say your name in a clear voice.

11. Treat fame and failure in the same manner, with indifference, for tomorrow is just another day.

✗✗✗✗✗✗✗

As a pharmacist, Papa was the best one I ever met. There was nothing he couldn't do. In the way of compounding prescriptions, I never saw him stumped. So it was with great surprise that I learned that he was not a registered pharmacist. In his day, it was sufficient and acceptable to do a long apprenticeship under a registered pharmacist. This my father did under his dad. So he was considered by the state a registered pharmacist. In the early 1930s they formed a pharmaceutical board, which held that apprentice pharmacists would be grandfathered in. This, Papa refused to do. Perhaps he never thought he would end up working as a pharmacist and needing a license again. Whatever the reason, he didn't apply to get his license through grandfathering. I attribute it to pure, old Spanish hard-headedness.

The shock of my life was to find that he had to work under another pharmacist's license. He couldn't run La Economica on his merits. I was shocked. It seemed like no one anywhere in Ybor City had legitimate documentation. The town's leading pediatrician Dr. Gavilla had turned out to be a naturopath, or a quack! Lawyers became lawyers by hanging around the courthouse. They never graduated from the university. Ybor City operated on the anarchy of a Banana Republic.

I learned how to manufacture all of types of drugs, from hard-to-make emulsions, to suppositories, pills, and powders. In our store we stocked old remedies from Cuba and Spain. We had a jar of leeches to suck blood out of a hematoma, also known as a black eye. I needed to reach in and put them in a Dixie cup. If they latched on to you, you had to burn them off with a cigarette, and I didn't smoke at all.

We dispensed every type of leaf, plant, roots, rhizomes, and gums, as well as the naturally available althea root, boric acid, seidlitz powders, and about 24 writers' natural drugs. That kept us busy manufacturing and packaging all day.

We had to continually sweep and dust the counters, for a fine dust storm swept into the open doors coating the bottles and displays. This, and a continuous battle with flies, was the duty of the delivery boy. Flies were taken care of by hanging strips of flypaper from the neon lights.

By 11 p.m. we were exhausted. The night watchman *(El Sereno)* would come to buy a 35-cent bottle of Bay Rum, an aftershave lotion, which he would open and drink right down in front of me. If Papa was around, the night watchman went outside, away from my father's stern gaze, and then drank it down.

Then we closed the store, got into our spiffy 1941 Chevy, and drove to the Columbia, where we would feast on a Cuban sandwich split in two and a *cafe con leche*. Then we jointly worked a crossword puzzle in the street edition of the *Tampa Tribune*. If we did not feel sleepy enough to go home, we drove out to the Sea Breeze Restaurant to hunt rabbits. We never caught any that I can remember. Were there rabbits behind the See Breeze? Or was Papa just running a gag on me? I never found out.

Then we went to a warm home. I was satisfied that somehow I contributed to the health and happiness of my father and that I pleased him and made him proud of me. Sleep came easy then.

An Innocent Affair

In every young boy's life there is a first love. The love bug bites early. The tyke smitten with love for another, though, doesn't know what is happening to him, nor what to do about it.

I was no different, but it was a long-standing, ongoing affair for years. What was odd about it was that it was distinctly unilateral. Only one side knew about it.

In my family, and in the neighborhood I played in, there were no females. We didn't have them, didn't need them. The closest thing you could call love, or an unnatural affection, was for a teacher. Mine was my third grade teacher, Mrs. Camel. She was a beautiful, kind, loving woman. I was two years ahead of my class, so I had to be protected. Mrs. Camel made my passage through third grade a safe and happy journey. Could you call what I felt for her love? No, I don't think so. It was more like the love I had for my maiden Aunt Lola who lived next door and spoiled me rotten. Affection, yes. Love, no.

At that age, you really have no idea of who you are. Are you tall? Skinny? Good looking or ugly? Fair? Dark? Tan? Is your hair nice? None of these things mattered to me. I was normal. Like everyone else. The only thing that set me apart was my clothes. My mother, an excellent seamstress, made my clothes. Boy, was that an embarrassment. Everybody had T-shirts and overalls from Sears. I looked like Prince Andrew. Looks are misleading, however. Although I looked like a rich kid, in actuality, my mother made my clothes from Papa's old suits, so the cost of our school clothes was zero. We looked rich and lived poor.

My long-standing fruitless, naïve love affair started in the seventh grade. We had graduated from Robert E. Lee Grammar School to Thomas Jefferson Junior High School. Most of our seventh grade class came over from Robert E. Lee. A few were new.

One of the new kids was Joyce Brantley. She was in my homeroom, and I sat right behind her. At first I was struck dumb by her beauty, her perky personality, and her intelligence. She wasn't high faluting. She didn't act good looking. And once she noticed me. She treated me well. This was because we were two years apart. The gap never shortened. When we finished junior high, she was 15 years old. I was still lagging way back at 13. This, you understand, did not diminish my infatuation; it increased it. A hopeless infatuation.

Then came high school, and Joyce exploded on all fronts. Beauty queen, ROTC sponsor, cheerleader, academic leader, school paper, annual committee, etc. Where there was a job to be done, she volunteered or was drafted. The entire school loved Joyce. Yet, she never went steady with a boy, nor dated very much. Most of this was because she needed to work nights to help support a dysfunctional family.

I had taken to waiting outside her house on Jefferson Street and Columbus Drive and kind of naturally fell in with her. We talked about homework and some school gossip, but never an acknowledgement of our friendship. Still, it was enough to walk her to school. I had a blissful relationship with Joyce. I made her laugh. I carried her books when she let me; I brought her extra chocolate milk at lunch and in general looked out for her. She thought my slavish attention was funny and sweet. That was all I could expect.

As we hit our senior year, I was struck—full force by what I now call Ferdie's Folly. I had never felt so completely enthralled by one girl. (In the interest of accuracy, I should point out that the exception is my wife, Luisita, my life-mate whom I decided to marry after our first date. But I was 43 years old then, and a seasoned womanizer. With Joyce, she had no competition.) The apex, the top of Ferdie's Folly, came when Joyce took a job as a cashier at the Florida Theatre, then called the Franklyn Theatre.

I figured Joyce had to get to work by taking the Jefferson streetcar, which passed right by my house. By running home, I could bathe, change, and be on her streetcar. The object of my affection would be on the car, I would sit next to her and have her all to myself, one on one, for the 15 minutes or so it took to get there. Now, mind you, I saw Joyce from morning until 3 p.m. at school every day, but I could never catch her alone. She attracted crowds. No sir, the Jefferson streetcar would be the answer!

Foolish as this sounds, looking at it 60 years later, I can tell you I stuck to my dogged scheduled for an entire senior year.

And *not once,* did I see Joyce on the streetcar. Infatuation occludes reason. By this time Joyce was 18 and a full-blown woman. A beauty. The town in 1944 was filled with pilots, second lieutenants with wings, pocketfuls of cash, and Ford convertibles. Streetcars? Joyce had a ride coming and going.

We graduated in June 1944. Most of our class was either in or going into the service. I was 16 and was going to go to medical school. I started at the University of Tampa, and quickly transferred to the University of Tennessee. After a brief stop there, I landed at Spring Hill College, a Jesuit penitentiary by the bay in Mobile, Alabama. I did very well there for three years.

In my senior year—I was 20 then—I was home for Christmas. I'd had a great Christmas break and went to meet my gang at the Big Orange. To my surprise, I ran into Joyce Brantley! She was in a car with her date, drinking hard. What a pleasant surprise. I had almost forgotten her. Quickly she told me of her last few years, how she married a Jefferson kid, divorced him, picked up a drinking problem, and was very successful on the job. She was the superintendent at the phone company. A pretty big job. She was a big success. So then…

"You are available?" I asked.

"Sure," she said and got out of the car and hugged me.

Rapidly, I made the date for the next night. I was leaving the following day and could have one last night with my beloved Joyce. Hot dog!

That day was spent in frantic activity. I washed and waxed the 1941 Chevrolet. I steam-cleaned my tan, gabardine suite (from Wolf Brothers), bought a fresh tie, filled the car with gas, took a fifth of scotch from the family liquor supply, made a reservation at the Sea Breeze. Joyce got off at 10 p.m. The Sea Breeze allowed you to eat until

1 a.m. or 2 a.m., and carry your bottle in, and then—and then, the empty beaches to ourselves. Hot dog! By then, the age difference had blurred. I was a man at 20, and the playing fields were leveled. In addition, Joyce had shown a great joy at seeing me. That was a headstart, for sure. This was it! The main event!

The day flew by fulfilling all of my tasks. But what to do between 6 p.m. and 10 p.m.? Those hours would be nerve-wracking and long!

Basketball! The University of Tampa had a fine basketball team, and they were playing the top team on the schedule, nationally ranked Louisville. I would go with my buddy, John Ranon, he in his car, me in mine, and I would leave at 9:30 p.m. no matter what the score.

Parking was impossible and cost one dollar. I was always a scofflaw, so I found that there was a traffic station on Northern Boulevard, right in front of Fort Homer Histerly Auditorium. Behind it was an empty lot with a big No Parking sign on it. Disregarding the sign, I parked and went in.

As good as the game was I could not get interested because Joyce would be waiting at 10 p.m. in front of the phone company. Wild horses couldn't keep me from my date at the appointed hour.

The night was ice cold. Frosted breath inside the car was good news. She'd have to snuggle close to me as we rode to the Seabreeze. This was going to be heaven!

I put the key in the ignition, the six-cylinder GM motor clicked over. No trouble. I put the car in reverse and gave 'er the gas.

But then, my heart sank along with the car, in the soft Florida sands of that back lot! And nothing can save you from soft sands but a wrecker.

I tried letting the air out of the tires and digging a trench out with my hands. Nothing. The car dug in deeper and deeper and deeper.

I was frantic. If I ran to the phone company, a good mile and a half, I wouldn't make it. There were no phones to call her. No house would open its door to let a sweaty, sandy young man in to use the phone. Nothing. Nothing. Nothing.

I was screwed by fate, not Joyce!

The trip back to Mobile was hell. I was disconsolate. There was no way to rectify my horrible behavior. I, a lowly serf, had stood up the queen—the greatest girl in the universe. How could I ever explain this? I didn't have any mailing address or phone number for Joyce. We might as well have lived on different planets.

Eventually, I sought solace in the arms of my steady girlfriend in Mobile, and slowly Joyce faded from memory. It took a couple of years.

When I got back for summer break, I found Joyce had married another Jeffersonian and was busily raising a boy and a girl. Well, *that* definitely closed *that* chapter.

Many, many years later, with me happily married to Luisita, with a beautiful daughter of my own, Tina, I was taken with the desire to write about growing up in Tampa. I published long pieces in the *Tampa Tribune* and *La Gaceta*. I wrote a long piece about streetcars and how I missed them and loved them.

One part of the story dealt with the fact that streetcars were not suited to love affairs. And remembering my Ferdie's Folly chasing Joyce, I wrote it up, with a glowing description of Joyce.

The reaction was outstanding and shocking!

I received a long letter from Vernell Davis, Joyce's sister-in-law. She informed me of the shocking news that Joyce had died! Burned up in bed! Drinking and smoking had brought about her untimely end. I was crushed! What sad news!

The purpose of the letter was to thank me for painting such a positive picture of Joyce as a young woman. How beautiful she had been. How smart. How popular. In short, a glowing picture of a queen.

Her children had only known her as an embarrassment. My heart bled for these kids, and so I wrote them a long letter describing Joyce when she was Queen of the Universe. Alcoholism is a disease, I explained, just like tuberculosis or cancer. It kills. Joyce was a victim. I think it helped them to see her through my adoring eyes.

Then the closure I sought came to me at the Jefferson 60th anniversary reunion. I sat talking to an old friend, the charming Dee Dee Roop. Suddenly, from left field, she said, "You know, I had lunch with Joyce the day after you didn't show up for your date."

Dee Dee recounted the conversation.

"You want to hear something strange?" Joyce had said. "Guess who stood me up for a supper date last night?"

"Who?" Dee Dee had asked.

"Ferdie Pacheco. My little pal did not show up. I wonder why?"

Well, now Joyce might get the message from the next Jeffersonian who makes it through the Pearly Gates.

Unexpected Detour:
The Prank that Cost Five Years

After a short time at the University of Tennessee where I had been initiated into Sigma Phi Epsilon, a social fraternity—heavy emphasis on social—my father decided I was having too much fun. He couldn't prove it. I was too sharp to be caught 1,000 miles from Ybor City. Still my father knew. In his bones, he knew. He decided that I had to leave Tennessee, attend Spring Hill College with my brother as a roommate, and study biology under a tyrant, Father P.H. Yancey.

The three years I spent being a Yancey top boy netted me a professorship, teaching mammalian anatomy laboratory, which consisted of dissecting alley cats. I got paid in cash and prestige. I had the privilege and trust of getting Father Yancey's keys to the lab, therefore, to his office. I was also on the basketball team; I wrote, painted, cartooned, and did comedy. In other words, by my senior year I was a B.M.O.C. (big man on campus).

The thing that saved my sanity was the admission of the returning war vets in 1946. This was an unholy lot of combat-fatigued, wounded, maimed, and thoroughly exhausted young men, who showed up primarily to collect their GI Bill. The Jesuits had no idea how to handle them, so they opened the gates and allowed them to go free into the night. The good part was the rest of the student body went with them.

At this point, luck, which had always been on my side, went over to the other side full time.

At the end of four years, before you could graduate, Father Yancey insisted on an oral comprehensive exam. Now, no one in the world could pass that exam. Not in biology. Not with fire-breathing Father Yancey giving you the third degree and the evil eye. On the other hand, no one had ever failed the test, either. So how hard could it be? I didn't even bone up. I was the No. 1 boy, professor of the mammalian anatomy lab. He couldn't flunk me. Yancey had hinted that he already had me accepted at Georgetown Medical School, in Washington D.C.

We had taken to driving down the Foot-Of-The-Hill Inn, where the beer was cold and the burgers were thick and out of this world. Money was no longer a problem, because GIs seemed to have plenty to spend. We had had a few, when the grisly master sergeant joined us and began to wail loudly about his inability to pass the comprehensive exam. (Now Sarge had been with the big red one and had made all of the invasions from North Africa to Sicily-Anzio and, finally, D-Day at Utah Beach. To say he was shaky was an understatement.) None of the wise-guy college students was worried, and we tried to reassure him, but the more we tried, the worse he cried.

Finally a few beers later, I got a bright idea. I had the key to Yancey's office. Yancey was away in St. Louis for the week. Father Mullahy, an obese Jesuit who didn't miss a meal, would be at dinner. Why not nip up to Yancey's office and steal the comprehensive exam? It seemed like a solution to me. We all agreed that one other boy, an A student named Peyton, would come with me.

Since the GIs got to Spring Hill, stealing the exams was a given. After all, many of the GIs had been OSS operatives. If they could break into German headquarters to steal papers, they'd certainly have no trouble with the innocent Jesuits.

Peyton was in Yancey's office having no luck finding the comprehensive exam when the unthinkable happened. Father Mullahy, the glutton, had left the dining room before dessert had been served and came by the biology lab to pick up his Parker pen.

It was semidark when I almost ran head on in to the rotund father.

"What are you doing here?" I blurted out.

"I'm looking for my pen. I left it here," he said, thoroughly confused by my presence in the darkened lab.

"That's my excuse," I said truthfully. I had semi-prepared an excuse if I was caught.

Hearing a commotion in the lab at that moment Peyton's voice from inside Yancey's office rang out.

"Who's out there?" he said in a loud whisper.

Caught, dead on, heart stopper, dead.

"Go to your rooms," said a confused Father Mullahy.

Two A students in one snare. What the hell?

Getting into a gigantic screw-up like that is a wonderful learning experience. You find out quickly that you are alone in this world. No one wants to be seen with you lest there be guilt by association. Priests scurry away from you lest they have to show empathy, pity, forgiveness, or any of those good things they read about in the Bible but fail to exercise in public.

I stayed isolated in my room, waiting for the disciplinary counsel sentencing. There was to be no hearing. The Jesuits, when they sniff guilt, get their blood up, and there is hell to pay.

The verdict was expectedly harsh. Expulsion, of course; marked in your transcript, for life, in red ink. If any medical school sent for a transcript or if Spring Hill ever heard you were applying to another school, they would send on the red ink transcript with a letter.

I could not accept so harsh and vindictive a punishment from men of the cloth. I asked to see the president.

The president was a young, early 40s ball of fire who had progressive ideas and had a reputation for fairness. Physically he looked like a young Abe Lincoln. He was fair. He listened sympathetically. Then, when all I had to say was said, he lowered the boom, sympathetically, as the Inquisitions Disciplinary Council had done. In effect, he rubber-stamped the verdict.

"Father, from my window every day for the past three years I see Jesuits, young and old walking down the paths between the pine trees," I said. "They seem to be deep into reading their Bibles."

"Yes, that is our hour to read and meditate."

"Yes, but, how many times can you read the same passages of the Bible before your mind goes blank. Can anyone on earth read a book 100 times? Don't you think they'd get the message pretty soon? Or do you think it is possible the message becomes a blank and eventually disappears?"

"What do you mean?" he straightened out in his high-backed chair sniffing out an insult hovering into view.

"I mean did you read the part about pity, Christian charity, and forgiveness? Didn't Christ, even in pain on the cross, say, 'Forgive them for they know not what they do?'"

"Yes, but this deals with college students in a university setting. There are rules to be obeyed."

"So, Christ didn't mean us? He had an exception put in the Bible. Forgive me I've only read the Bible once, but I didn't see anywhere, in the Bible where it said, *'Except for college students.'*"

"Well, we have a school to run."

"Much more important than the world to run as Jesus had, I'm sure."

I got up to leave because I knew I was toast.

"Father this verdict is vindictive. They mean to keep me from becoming a doctor by excessive and restrictive means. I won't have it. I'll get it changed. And in the end, I'll become a doctor."

I was getting hotter, he, more glacial, aloof, and withdrawn.

Then in an ill-timed, ill-advised exit remark I said, "And by the way, of those who judged me so harshly one is a pederast whom I confronted in the confessional and the other an open homosexual. Neither man wants anything good to happen to me. Look to your own house, Father, and judge the greater crimes being committed here. And those *are* in the Bible."

Of course, that was in 1948, when Jesuits caught engaging in homosexuality, pederasty, sodomy, or larceny were not turned over to the authorities but were either transferred to another parish or, if the crime was large enough, were sent to permanent exile to Grand Châteaux in Louisiana, a Jesuit Devil's Island for wayward priests.

Either way my ill-advised comments fell on deaf ears, because in those days no priest would acknowledge these crimes of their fellow men of God. Good priests closed their eyes and prayed harder that all would go away.

I still had to undergo my greatest ordeal. I had to confront Father Yancey, my patron, the man who had trusted me and positioned me to go to medical school. How badly I had treated him! I had accepted his trust and befouled it by an unspeakable act. What was worse than anything was that there was no motive for this senseless crime. We were trying to help someone else. Neither the other kid nor I had had any worries about passing the comprehensive exam.

Great was the tongue lashing I was in for. And well deserved, too. That was step one of my agony. Step two, was worse, I would have to face my broken-hearted father, who was willing himself to stay alive, just so he could see me a graduate as a doctor. So far, things had been acceptable, now came hell.

With tears running down my cheeks I trudged up the three flights of creaky old wooden steps of the new biology hall, my hands in my pockets, feeling like I had a 100-pound weight on my back, my heart was heavy with embarrassment and sadness. If Yancey had hit me over the head with a baseball bat, I would have thanked him.

Patrick Henry Yancey was about 55 years old at the time. His body was wide and sturdy. His face was patrician. He was balding down the middle of his head, and the sides were abundant and gray. He had a small, cruel thin-lipped mouth and dingy teeth. He was fearsome, but I was not afraid of him; after all I spent almost every day of three years working at his side. He had treated me like a son.

I pulled myself together and opened the door. He was seated quietly at his desk, where a small green shaded light was the only illumination in the room. His hands were tented, his head was down, his eyes studied his green blotter.

I said nothing, took my chair directly in front of him, and folded my arms.

A long moment of silence then ensued. Only our heavy breathing was heard. Then Father Yancey started to talk in his quiet whispering way, like a Mafia don.

"Where did I fail you? This accident is my entire fault. If I had not made the comprehensive exam seem so difficult to pass, this would not have happened. You two boys have been through the worst, toughest classes I could teach." He began to sob. "Do you really think I would base four years of hard work on one exam?

"Ferdie, you should have known. There is no comprehensive exam! I just have tea and chat about the student's future, there was no exam to steal."

He fell silent as the enormity of my stupidity dawned on me. He had conned all of the seniors into a gigantic, six-week review cram session. This refreshed what we had needed to know and showed us how to handle big-time pressure. That was the Yancey method!

"All of my life in teaching I've been wrong!" he said. "How many good boys flunked out because of me? Had they gone to the University of Alabama, they might have made As and gotten into schools. I thought if I made premed tougher than medical school I would have done my duty. None of my boys has ever flunked out. But what about the ones who deserved the chance, and I denied them that chance?"

Well, he had a point there. Many good, average kids did not make it to medical school because of Yancey, and I was about to be one more. Then, he seemed to shuck off his self-pity and blame-taking and came back to the old solve-the-problem Yancey I knew.

"First of all Ferdie, you can forget all of the revengeful, spiteful rules of the disciplinary committee. I threw that verdict out. They had no jurisdiction over a Yancey boy, much less my No. 1 boy. You will have nothing on your record. You pulled out because of reasons of family health. Period. Not a word of anything else."

I wondered what the president had thought when he heard Yancey's pronouncement. Perhaps now he knew the Lord moves in strange ways. Perhaps, there was an exception to his exception in the Bible.

The look of relief on my face must have seemed so evident that it gave Yancey heart.

"Do you have a place to go hide out for a week?"

He sounded like a co-conspirator.

"Yes, sir. My buddy Larry Guerra is in Dental Tech's School in New Orleans, just married. He'll take me in."

"Good. Go there and try to put this aside."

"What aside?"

I was tempted to wise-guy it but thought the better of it.

"When you get home, have a plan for your future. Your dad, J.B., will not mention it again. You don't either. Just go ahead with your plan. I regret not counting you in my graduating Yancey's boys, but I am sure you will get into medical school, and you will be a great doctor."

✗✗✗✗✗✗

After seven days of eating well and listening to New Orleans jazz, I appeared at my home in Tampa in time for breakfast.

Papa was shaving with his Gillette two-way razor in the white tiled bathroom. I came in, felt silly trying to kiss his cheek because it was all lathered, and took my customary seat on the rim of the oversized tub.

"What are you going to do now?" he asked.

"I'm going to pharmacy school. I hear it is very important to get into medical school if you have a professional degree. I should be able to do pharmacy in one year, since I have 140 hours of credits, enough for a degree in biology, chemistry, English, history, and, thanks to the Jesuit requirements, philosophy."

"That sounds good."

Mindful of the horrible expenses he had endured with my four years at a private school and my brother's annual psychotic breakdowns, I tried to lighten the load.

"The tuition at Florida is $50 a semester if you'll take care of that, I'll take care of the rest ($50 for room and board). I know how to make money in college, so I'll pay for it all."

The problem came when I found out that they had just passed a state law, which said it took three years to complete a degree in pharmacy. There followed two years in the Air Force, because the Korean War was on. What a waste of time that was.

If you are counting, that prank cost me five years before I got into medical school. Oddly enough, I never thought that I wouldn't get in and never thought that I wouldn't become a doctor. I just accepted the fact that I'd done something dumb, and I had to pay the price. There's a lesson to be learned. Persistence pays, but never quit, never!

A Platonic Affair

The fall semester at the University of Florida had started in 1950 with the same mild disappointment, the loss of the first football game. By this time, I had been in a college for seven years, chasing an impossible admission into medical school and failing that, getting a degree in pharmacy. Ugh.

I was bored. Played out. It was the same old routine. School was now co-ed. Thousands of great looking, freshmen girls flock to Gainesville. Easy pickings. Too easy. No challenge. No real entertainment, except for easy sex, and the complications that brings.

The first week the university got all of the fraternities and sororities to throw a huge public street dance. Just simply that. A good d.j., a wide-open circle, and cold drinks. It was packed, and a great way to review the pickings. Lots of babes.

Early in the evening I spotted a gorgeous girl. The big mop of ginger blond hair, waving seductively as she danced. Her figure was eye-popping, although fashions that year had dropped the hemlines to the ankle, and full fuzzy sweaters obscured the bust line. My eyes stayed riveted on this beautiful girl with the wild hair and the knockout body. She slid smoothly, not missing a beat or a shake of the hips, or a shrug of the shoulder. She was hot. I stay glued to her all night, all but tongue-tied at intermission. She did not notice me or even give me a nod. When the dance was over about 11 p.m., I decided to make my move, my never-fail bashful approach. I walked along beside her on the campus sidewalk.

"I would have liked to dance with you, but I couldn't bring myself to ask you." I mumbled my head down.

"Why didn't you?"

She smiled a very friendly smile, kind of teasing, yet open and inviting.

"You dance too good. I don't know how to bop, and you are the best I've seen."

"You don't have to bop to dance with me, I like slow dancing, and I dance to all Latin music. Don't sell yourself short." She smiled a slow, easy, stunning smile.

"I was just thinking of you. I didn't want to embarrass you." I stammered badly.

"So what? Does this mean you'll never ask me, never? Ever never?"

She was toying with me. This was no child student girl. I saw that she was about my age, 24 or 25, a grown woman. No ring on her finger. She might be in the same shape as me: an old student in the midst of the young chickadees.

"I'll learn to bop if you teach me this week, and by Friday I'll dance every dance."

We had walked to the off-campus strip of food cafes. To my surprise and joy, I found she lived next to Dave's Diner in a big old Southern house that was an apartment for women. She put out her hand.

"Bette Swenson is my name. I'm a reporter for the *St. Pete Times*. I'm up here to do my nine months in journalism, graduate, and marry my fiance in June. We went together during the war. I waited for him until he was discharged, and then waited some more until he finishes his chiropractic training in June, and finally we're getting married."

"Puff, puff," I laughed at her long, one-breath sentence. "Getting married. At last."

"At last."

We were laughing together, as if she and I had just posted our boundaries. Now we knew where we were going, and where we were not going. It seemed so fresh and open and natural. We'd just met, but it felt like I had just concluded a good deal.

"Done deal," I said to myself.

That Friday night, we sat on the steps until 3 a.m. She brushed a near-miss kiss on my cheek, and I found myself blurting out, "What are you doing for breakfast?"

"Breakfast?"

She laughed at the absurdity of having breakfast with a boy she'd just met.

"I only have coffee and a doughnut," she said.

"That's fine; I only have a quarter, so it fits my wallet."

She squealed in delight. She was very down to earth, and money never posed a problem between us. She equated being broke with being funny. I didn't.

That night I lay in bed mesmerized by her electric personality and brilliant good looks. We had talked for hours, first me and my wacky stories, and then her and her newspaper stories. She really was a reporter. I was impressed. I barely slept until 8 a.m. When I walked over to her house, she was already sitting on the steps, this time in a T-shirt and white, starched tennis shorts. It turns out she was a tennis star as well, and she had perfect legs to prove it.

"I thought you weren't coming," she teased.

"If I was any earlier, we might as well have never said good night last night.

"Yeah. That was fun. You are really a great storyteller."

"Anybody from Ybor City is a storyteller."

"So I've heard."

Dave's Diner was one of a kind. Every college town has one. It was a no-nonsense diner, mostly hamburgers and "the best" hot dogs, soups, breakfasts, and pies in the world. Dave had a fatal weakness: He generally loved college kids. By mid-semester he was on a first-name friendship with each kid who ate there.

He had installed what he called the honor system. As a customer came in he picked a blank check. He was responsible for putting down what he ate, adding it up, and paying Dave on the way out. Dave knew danged well he got stiffed a lot, but he didn't care. Dave felt that the boy who didn't have money would come back eventually and repay him. I was never sure that worked, but it did with Bette and me. Some days we were both broke. Dave would just wave us on by. Bette and I always tried to pay him back. Dave never got rich on our money, but by the time he died, he was a wealthy man. He was beloved by generations of young kids, and that has a great deal of value.

We spent the entire day together, highlighted by going to a swimming pool. Bette had the kind of figure that you now see in *Sports Illustrated* bathing suit issues. In those days, white latex, one-piece bathing suits, à la Esther Williams, were the thing, and Bette stopped conversation in mid-sentence when she stepped off the high board in a perfect swan dive. I came to learn that she was a natural athlete.

Everything came easy to her. In those days I was a pretty good athlete myself, so we were well matched. And, yes, she was better than me in everything. One day, early in our talkathon, she came in with a quizzical look on her face.

"What's this I hear from the frat brothers about what a big, bad practical joker you are? What's up with that?"

"Oh, that. It's just a horrible fault I have. When I see guys who are assholes or puffed up, self-important buffoons, I like to do things to them to deflate them."

"Oh, that sounds like fun. But how to get away with it?"

"That's the first lesson. Nobody reacts like they should. There's never any anger. The bigger the gag, the less anyone reacts."

"I'd love to see that."

"Listen, you are a drama student, so acting is easy. Second, you have a minor in psychology, so you can guess how this is going to go. Are you ready?"

"Just tell me what to do."

I was in heaven, for it's hard to get beautiful women to be part of stunts. Some find them embarrassing; some find them infantile. Bette found them fun.

"This Saturday get dressed as well as you can. Do your hair, nails, makeup, the full movie star shot. Wear your finest dress. We will go to the student center dining room. The place will be packed. We will attract attention just by our entrance."

She did exactly as I instructed and we arrived at the dining hall in style. When we came in, everyone looked at us. We sat down and began to eat. Then midway through the meal, we started to argue. First rumbles, then louder with some cuss words. As we finished the meal, we were shouting at each other. The manager was on his way over when Bette stood up, picked up a plate of lemon meringue pie, and said, "I'm not taking that from you."

She slammed the pie in my face.

"I am not taking that from you," I said before, of course, doing the same.

Our audience gasped, but no one moved for a long moment. Calmly, I looked at my wristwatch, and said, "Come, my dear, we'll have to hurry if we are going to make the beginning of the movie."

And we walked out, arm in arm.

There was stillness in the hall, and then the buzz of people discussing what they had just seen. Bette laughed as we headed for Dave's to wash our faces.

No prank was beneath Bette. Once, I bet a fraternity brother that Bette and I could make it to Miami (about 700 miles) with absolutely zero money in our jeans. We predicated our success on how good an actress Bette had become and what a fool the average man is for a good story from a spectacularly beautiful woman. That bet was a no-brainer. We got gas, oil, water, a loaf of white bread, a jar of Smuckers strawberry jam, a bar of cream cheese, and a six-pack of Coke. No problem— all she had to do was smile! Men are all suckers!

✗✗✗✗✗✗

The campus was filled with wonderful student activities. Once, Sir Laurence Melchior, the great Danish tenor, who had found a home in Esther Williams's films, came to sing for us. He was robust and full of fun. He was just getting warmed up when the whistle blew at 9 p.m., the signal for freshman girls to be in their dorms.

"Nonsense!" he yelled.

"Girls, go to your dorms, change into your p.j.s, and I'll be there to sing you to sleep. Go to your windows!"

They did, and he did.

True to his word, he got the boys to bring cases of beer, all on him, and he went to the girls' dorms, and sang his lungs out until midnight. What a lovely night. Bette loved it! We had a champion's season of entertainment for nine months. What fun!

Looking at those nine months of a lovely relationship, it seems impossible that we had such a close friendship without the monster *sex* rearing its ugly head. I put it in a category of a miracle. And maybe it was.

I'm not saying that we didn't stray from time to time and get into some heavy high school necking. We really dug each other, so why not? It wasn't going anywhere. South of the border, I mean.

Just when that premise looked shaky, Bette brought her kid brother, Ollie, to enroll in school. He was 10 years younger than us and brought a kind of puppy-dog lovability with him. To begin with, he worshipped Bette, who was like a hip mother to him. At first, he was kind of sullen around me. He couldn't understand how I fit in. Was I like a boyfriend? No, couldn't be, because Bette was engaged for Christ's sake. Bette, in her cool way, just let things simmer and explain themselves on their own. Soon Ollie understood, and he fit in perfectly. And, oh, by the way, he brought us independence in the form of a 1940 Ford convertible. Now that really expanded our pranks network. I also got Ollie rushed by my fraternity, Sigma Phi Epsilon, which being the senior member I called a Signal Foo Edelson to the consternation of the more serious brothers who were frankly at a loss to figure out my Bette-Ollie-Ferdie family.

This culminated in a grand-slam dunk of a prank. The more serious of the brothers, those who were at Gainesville to actually get an education and not there to dodge the draft and sweat out the Korean War, had been grumbling about our slovenly dress and our flaunting of dining room rules. We were a disgrace. Too loud. Too vulgar. Too shabbily dressed. They actually took a vote to make us dress well for guest night.

I went into immediate action with Bette's enthusiastic help. All of the boys were to wear white dinner jackets. Bette was to be our guest of honor. She dressed in a white formal strapless dress, did her hair up, and applied the movie star makeup. In short, Miss America stuff. We had chilled wine (a bucket at both ends of the table) to be served by four impeccably dressed waiters. We had a violinist playing pieces from operettas, and then, occasionally, swinging into a surprisingly exuberant Dixie, which obliged the entire dining room to stand singing in a loud voice.

✗✗✗✗✗✗✗

We were having a blast. But May came into view and with it the realization that we were going to graduate, and in June, we would part and our great and good friendship would dissolve and evaporate. Finito della comedia.

Fate and my innate good luck caused us to have one final act. We would not go away whimpering. We would go out with a bang. And what a bang!

Bette and I took one class together. It might have been the best class I ever took while in my entire 12-year career. The class was criminology. It was awesome, because it was taught by a true rogue professor, Dr. Vetter, who was in his 60s.

For his master's degree, Dr. Vetter had gone underground and rode the rails with the cutthroat bums of the rails. He had a better and much more dangerous idea for his doctorate. He got himself sentenced to 10 years in the toughest jail in America, Sing Sing. Only the warden knew it was a hoax. If anything had happened to the warden, Dr. Vetter faced 10 tough years. He found the only thing the cons really respected, and left you alone for, was to do time as a safe cracker. Safe crackers were the rock stars of the convict society.

Dr. Vetter looked like a Hollywood producer—tweed coat with leather elbow patches, white button-down shirts from Sy Dover in New York, and a wide black knit tie. Of course, he drove a 1949 Cadillac convertible, top down, always.

To add to his reputation as a hell-for-leather guy, that semester he scored a beautiful queen of a girl, the 17-year-old daughter of a full professor, and married her. How many did that make? He'd lost count.

Dr. Vetter organized a field trip to Raiford Penitentiary to visit two cons who were about to get the chair. Vetter announced to the class with some relish, as if he were announcing that Britney Spears was going to lap dance in your face, "Those of you with a nerve will have permission to sit in the electric chair. You will also have a 10-minute one-on-one interview with the cons about to die. I don't expect there will be many takers."

As expected, Bette was first in line. She still sent in stuff to the *St. Petersburg Times,* so a nice one-on-one with those about to be fried was right up her alley.

I passed on all that. Hell, I had a lot of friends out in the yard. Ybor City was well represented in the prison population. A couple of my old pals would soon visit the big chair, or if they got out, had a Mafia coming-out party ready to welcome them into oblivion.

Dr. Vetter gleamed with his approval. He loved us, and every time he talked to Bette, his eyes lit up in spite of having to take care of a 17-year-old beauty back home.

We had borrowed Ollie's car because he was a freshman and could not take criminology.

For the first time in three months, we were truly alone. A boy, a girl, a car, and a time to spare. Thank you, Dr. Vetter!

✗✗✗✗✗✗✗

The Florida sun was just starting to descend when we came to our first decision. The Raiford road came to a T-dead-end stop. Left, and we'd go back to Gainesville. Right, and we'd end up in St. Augustine, which neither one of us had ever seen but wanted to.

Of course, hidden agendas revolved around our heads. For example, if we went left, we faced the night together chaperoned by innocent Ollie. Also neither one of us had much money. Especially not enough for two rooms. Rapidly our choices were compressing us into a sort of delightful predicament. I was too scared to suggest what I was thinking. Not so for Bette, who seemed to take life in stride. After all, if you just spent 20 minutes talking to two young men about to die and leave this earth and all of its pleasures, a simple judgment call, like sharing a motel room with an old friend, ain't a big question, you know?

Bette just pointed east; I put the spunky convertible in first, put the top down, and roared off to our truly memorable night.

The Fort, the Room, and Other Memorable Parts

We pulled up to St. Augustine as they were closing the fort for the day. A thick, heavy rainstorm was heading our way. Bette shot into the main ranger's office, breathless with her supplication that we (two young lovers) from the university should be allowed to visit the fort. After all, she said we were studying the conquistadors and this was a perfect example of an old Spanish colonial fort.

He took one good look at her and my pleading face and said, "Okay, you got 15 minutes, and be careful the rain squall don't catch you, or you may never get out."

We went skipping around; the fort is really something to see and examine. We went to the top parapet. At each corner was a round turret, made snug and small to fit a solitary sentry.

The main guard came to escort us out but was driven back by a hauling, raging sheet of rain, lightning, and thunder.

Bette and I dove for the turret. We were getting soaked. Automatically we fell into a protective clinch. The turret was small, meant for a 15th-century Spanish shrimp, not two healthy American college kids. In all the time we had spent together, we never stood and hugged. There was a lot of good stuff in Bette to hug and hug and hug. The natural course of this, as you all have guessed by now, is a thundering kiss, with all the extras, French fries and onions.

A kiss eight months in the making is a powerful force of nature. It can't be held back. It can't be stopped. Both of us felt it to our toes. The rain continued. The warden came by decked out in his rain gear and viewed our heartfelt kiss with professional detachment.

"I'll give you 10 more minutes, or I'm calling in a minister to perform the wedding ceremony," he said with a good-natured laugh.

Thinking that we were closing in on a world record on foreplay, we dove out in the rain. "Boy," I thought, "if college students could just see history through our eyes, the fort would be a major attraction."

Correctly guessing that we were broke, our warden suggested an old broken-down Florida boarding house, on the shore, for our lodgings that night. It was closed for the season, but the old lady who ran it lived there and didn't mind an occasional boarder for the night. It was cheap, and for a reason—no electricity, no radio, no lights, one towel, and a set of fresh sheets for the night. But only one pillow for a double bed. Take it or leave it, $5. Perfect!

We found it. It looked like the house in Alfred Hitchcock's *Psycho*. It was battered and badly in need of paint. The shutters banged against the wall. The small light bulb lit the sign.

La Gondola
Closed for the Season
No vacancies, No Yankees

Skipping the formalities, Bette brazenly pushed the button. It took time, but a Florida shore bum of an old lady showed up holding a kerosene lamp.

"You the folks Ranger Elkins sent over?"

"Yes, ma'am," Bette said primly. I hung back, afraid to speak.

"The ones in heat?"

She cackled a sort of laugh. Bette looked down, acting embarrassed. I looked down too, but I *was* embarrassed.

She opened the door, and we followed the arc of dim light down the hall.

"I'm giving you my best room. Ocean view. You don't need air-conditioning if you open the windows. Sometimes after midnight you're going to get a present. Tonight is a full moon. The squall will have played out, and you're going to see one of nature's great sites. A full moon over the Atlantic Ocean after a storm. You fellers is lucky."

"That we are. Is there a place we can get something to eat?"

"Cheap," I added.

"I already fixed that. You walk about 100 yards to the right, bout as long as a football field. There you will see Captain Jim's Seafood Shanty. It ain't much. Years ago Captain Jim's boat floundered in a storm and come up here upside down. Hell, in them days nobody owed the shore, so Capt. Jim just let her set and one day, he got to fixing up the inside to feed a few people. He featured the catch of the day. He put out some lobster traps and caught delicious crabs, too. He found he could cook and liked to talk to strangers. So that's where you're going."

"Whoa, catch of the day don't sound cheap to me," I said, aware of our paucity of purse. "We got hamburger money."

"Did I say anything about money?" she repeated. "I said I'd called Capt. Jim, and he and I is splitting the cost. He got the better part of the deal. His fish and stuff ain't costing him nothing. Tomorrow he'll have to discard the fish, no how. I'll take your five dollars and buy you the finest red wine you ever tasted. Captain Jim makes it so it ain't costin' him nothing!"

"That sounds wonderful!" gushed Bette.

"Go on and git. That ol' fool don't like to be kept waiting even by the likes of a looker like you."

The overturned boat turned into a three-table restaurant looked like it came out of an MGM movie, *Treasure Island,* I figured. And Captain Jim was Wallace Barry without the parrot. A hearty-har-har type of guy.

"What happened to your parrot?" I wise-guyed.

"Had him for breakfast. He was very good with mustard." Har, har, har.

One small drawback. He loved to entertain by playing an accordion. Duke Ellington used to say that the definition of a gentleman is a man who knows how to play an accordion but won't. I heartily concur.

Notwithstanding the accordion, the food was to die for, a filet of grouper with the fixings and a full lobster for us—and dessert, key lime pie, of course.

The walk down the surf's edge was blissful. The waves crashed violently after the storm. The spray felt good. It was May, but the summer heat was on us. The spray cooled us off.

I don't know about Bette, but I was a tangle of nerves trying to figure out what to do about bedding for the night. There was definitely *not* anywhere but that *big* double bed. There was and then again, there wasn't a problem. Depending on if you were Bette or if you were Ferdie. The bed looked soft, but the floor was definitely hard and, in Florida, cockroaches own the floor and walls. I saw roaches the size of Buicks. Ugh. Not for me!

As usual Bette had the whole thing solved. She pulled her wet blouse and skirt off. They were wet, but her slip was not. She looked wonderful in the penumbral light of the kerosene lamp. Why, I wondered, did Edison invent electric light?

"Take your wet clothes off," she said and got under the covers. Her abundant hair spread over the one pillow.

Of course, I did not have the advantage of a covering slip. When my shirt and pants came off, I was left in my GI BVDs and nothing else. Not even an undershirt. I lay down on top of the covers because I couldn't in all consciousness get under the covers in just BVDs. The spring night had turned chilly, and the breeze off the ocean was brisk and chilly.

Bette, smiling at my discomfort, pulled the covers up and invited me in.

"Come on, you dope, get in. It's cold. And I'm not going to bite you."

After what felt like an eternal period of time, we rolled over toward one another, hugged, and finally picked up our volcanic kiss where we had left off. I can only report that we never got around to the big L, but the night flew by in intense delight, stuck to each other by mutual need and enjoyment. Dawn arrived, and we were still glued together. We slept an hour or so, got up, dressed, and headed out for Gainesville and Dave's Diner for our 20-cent breakfast.

What had happened? Nothing and yet everything. We didn't talk, overanalyze it, examine it, nothing. We just knew we were perilously close to disaster. But somehow we averted it. Why was I thankful? Was she? I think so. I hope so.

Graduation and endings were always embarrassments to me. I couldn't seem to do endings well, either.

After four years of very hard productive work on a premed degree, biology, and chemistry, I was tossed out by the Jesuits SS with four weeks left until graduation. Granted it was a stupid stunt. I was at fault. I never asked for pity. I just shouldered the blame and soldiered on. But it set me back five years, and it hurt badly.

At Florida I had accumulated enough hours for the degrees in biology, chemistry, English, history, and philosophy, yet I never went to pick them up. Never went to graduations. Meaningless paper to me. I never even told my family.

I wanted a pharmacy degree as a method of getting into medical school. I thought the schooling was stupid and wildly unnecessary. Still, I needed that paper.

We were graduated one hot June day. Everyone at the fraternity house was overwhelmed by joy. The end of the road. The beginning of life. Hooray!

My poor dad, a man easily a king in his surroundings, was pathetically out of place at graduation. He'd bought a new suit. The first in 20 years. I always saw him in dark blue suits. This time some haberdasher who owed him money tried to pay him back by giving him a new suit. It was a bilious green suit horribly out of place on my poor old conservative, dignified father. In Ybor City he was a king. In Gainesville he looked like a clown.

He came with his best friend, Frank Alonso, who was a great politician, always at home no matter where he was. I wanted Papa to meet Bette and Ollie and their St. Pete relatives, but Frank correctly sized up the situation. Papa felt so embarrassed and ashamed, so we slipped out of town hurriedly as if we had robbed the Wells Fargo Bank.

CHAPTER 3

Tough Goodbyes

Paula: Tragic Love

I expected the worse; I got the best. Well, next to the best. My college roommate had assured me that the two sisters were beautiful and fun. I was doubtful. I hated blind dates. Besides, I was already engaged to an Alabama beauty, in Mobile, and could not see any need to spend a night making idle chatter with a total stranger. To add to my pessimism, the two sisters were daughters of the juvenile judge, a fact that did not hold great promise.

I got the older one, at my request. As a world-wise 20-year-old college senior, I could not see myself with a 16-year-old high school girl. I met my date on the porch of an old rambling Florida house. I started to smile at my good luck. She was tall, an abundant amount of red hair attractively framed a pretty face, with milk white skin and highly freckled. She was beautifully proportioned with ample breastworks, a trim waist, and long legs. Scarlett O'Hara. I'd won the Belle o' the South lottery.

I hardly paid attention to my roommate's date until we got into the lights of the downtown streets. If I'd gotten Scarlett, then my pal had drawn Ava Gardner. She was slim and tall. Where Scarlett looked like a daughter of the South, her sister looked like a sophisticated, international model. Her hair was jet black, her eyes sparkled, and her high cheekbones set off her eyes in a spectacular fashion. A fine, perfectly proportioned nose seemed to point to a beautiful full mouth. Her chiseled chin led to a long, graceful neck.

Electricity jolted my senses. Her personality dominated the four-some. Her smile lit up the room. Her eyes crinkled when she smiled, and she was easy to make laugh, seeming to enjoy every story, to partake in every conversation. This young beauty had a brain! When we went to dance, I found a perfect partner in her. My date was good, but the younger girl sizzled when she danced. I could not take my eyes off of her when she danced. She was built for grace and movement. Her long legs were shapely, perfect, pretty legs. I found myself directing my attention and my conversation to this exciting beauty. My date did not seem to mind, almost as if she were used to this reaction on double dates.

The evening ended, and we bid our good nights on the screen porch. I made a mental note to call my friend's date—her name was Paula—first thing in the morning, because my roommate was going off to Georgetown Medical School and I to the University of Florida Pharmacy School.

There appeared to be a tremendous advantage to life at Gainesville, and that was its proximity to Tampa. I did anything I could to make money to be able to go home every weekend to see her. Those weekends were heaven for me, and soon the memories of my Alabama fiancée faded into obscurity, and I quit writing to her, and soon the engagement withered and died.

During this time of hot physical attraction, we were as one, happy in our mutual lustful attraction. She was daring, willing to take chances, to defy her father and his curfews. Her sister began to go with my best friend, and the happy times rolled on. Football games, frolics in fall and spring, and many weekends at home habituated me to the stunning beauty and her fun-filled ways.

On Sundays, with the weekend ending, with a hot and feverish Saturday night to recover from, we would go to the Centro Español and dance the remaining hours away, ending the evening, tired and soaked with perspiration, by dancing to the sign-off last tune, a Glenn Miller arrangement of "Adios." All week my senses would relive that final dance, because it was this dance that brought everything together. The smell of her hair, her makeup, the feel of her breasts against my chest, my leg pressing against her perfect thighs, encased in a smooth silk dress, and her arms around my neck, her head on my shoulder, looking up from time to time so I could drink from her full, luscious lips. It was a sensual perfection.

Eventually, I knew, this would come to an end, as all of my rela-tionships had done.

So, in time, she went her way and I was left to try to forget her, as I had all of the other beauties that had occupied my college years. Some had been harder to forget than others, but this one became an exception. She was irretrievably enmeshed in my memory. For the first time in my life I dreamed of her. Sleep did not come easily, and I relived my amorous moments with her, the sweet moments at the matinees, the aphrodisiac strains of "Adios," and the silk skirt rubbing against her thighs and pressing into me as we twirled, time suspended for a few moments, as if these moments had to last us for days and days of separation.

My days that spring were a nightmare I had never experienced before. I had always been able to forget one girl by finding a better one—or in the soothing practice of promiscuity. But because I knew that the attraction was more than physical, more than erotic, I knew I was doomed to longtime agony. I knew she had conquered my soul. The truth was I loved her company, loved to be in her presence. To be with her, no matter where we were. The pride I felt in being with the crowning beauty was childish and immature. I had always worshipped beauty, and she was my idea of perfection, but I knew that that was not it. Defined in any way, the fact was I was irrevocably in love with the gorgeous girl with the devilish eyes. And the worse part was that it was not going away, not being lessened, but sinking in, deep in my gut, solid and permanent like a slab of marble.

Fall brought the bad news that she was enrolling at Florida State University. So near, yet so far.

As I knew it would, spring brought the worst news: She was getting married. Who was the guy? He was from a well-to-do Tampa family. His family was in the food broker business, and her family knew the boy's family. They were respectable, fairly wealthy, and dull.

How could this most excellent girl settle for that inadequate boy? Would he appreciate what he had? Would he venerate her perfection? Could that electric mind of hers settle in as a young matron of Tampa's stodgy, uninventive, dull society? Could she stand it?

Obviously not!

I graduated that summer; she had a baby girl and divorced the dull food broker. The Korean War was heating up, and I faced armed forces duty unless I stayed in school. The combination of these factors resulted in my enrollment at the University of Tampa to complete work on English and history degrees.

It seemed inevitable that we would take up our steaming affair and that it would seem as if the intervening two years of anguish and pain had never happened, and that this was a continuing phase of our romance.

The big-screen porch of her house on Nebraska Avenue now held a playpen, and the beautiful baby now played contentedly on the lap of her grandmother and grandfather, aunts and uncles, and her mother's fiancé, for so I had become, almost without declaration or announcement.

The Air Force could not be put off any longer, and in the summer I faced another protracted period of pain. I signed up for four years and went in as a corporal in spite of my professional status and degrees. She had experienced great success as a model that year and felt that she should try her luck in New York, in the big time. So a deal was made. I would get two months of basic training out of the way; she would move into the Barbizon Hotel and try the bright lights. The baby would stay with her folks.

At the end of basic training, she came, riding up from Tampa with my parents. The tune playing everywhere that fall was Patti Page's "See the Pyramids Along the Nile…"

All I could do was hold on to her. She seemed equally happy to share our time, and almost without further conversation we got married. She had satisfied her curiosity about New York and a career in modeling, and I had found a partner to make the four years of the Air Force bearable and to share the rest of my life with.

So we loaded a U-Haul trailer with her household goods. The baby's mattress was strapped on to the roof of our new 1951 Chevrolet four-door car, and we set off for our new life.

✗✗✗✗✗✗

San Antonio now seemed a wondrous place to me as I took her to the great steak restaurants and enjoyed the Riverwalk and the clubs available on the air base. On the way to Texas we had stopped to visit New Orleans and the French Quarter. After the two months of deprivation I felt a sudden exhilaration, as if I had been reborn, when I, in a new tan Palm Beach suit, saw her in a freshly pressed white linen suit and the baby in her pinafore. We rediscovered the joys of the Court of the Two Sisters and walked the narrow streets of the quarter. Unmindful that we were stretching the budget to its breaking point, we started our married life, as we intended to live it, in first class.

Before we could settle into a routine we were transferred to El Paso and a S.A.C. base, Biggs Air Force Base. Once again we loaded our goods into the U-Haul and headed for a new adventure. We were lighter by one mattress, having lost it on the way from Tampa to San Antonio.

El Paso, Texas, in 1952, was by any measure, awful. A primitive border town across the Rio Grande from Juarez, it was actually a desert town. It was dry and hot, and a slight wind would stir up a dust storm. Grit was the main ingredient. It got in your clothes, on your furniture, and in your teeth.

We were oblivious of the discomfort. We were oblivious to our precarious financial position. Our rent was $120 a month, and my salary was $160 a month. Obviously a prescription for financial ruin.

Before we were ensconced in a modest garage apartment, we both found extra jobs, she as a model at the only big and local department store, I at the Fulton Drugstore.

It was during this period that I discovered an even greater perfection in my bride. She was resilient. She was a child of the South. Southern women, of large families, have a great sense of survival, of pulling their weight, of making do, of putting a good face on things, and of a great lack of self pity. As long as the family was together, everything was okay. Coming up in the ancient Spanish tradition of the man being the provider, I was surprised at her toughness.

She got up, fixed a hardy breakfast, bathed and dressed the baby, and then prepared herself as the reigning beauty queen of El Paso. I took the baby to the base nursery and reported for duty. When I returned to the tiny apartment with the baby, she was already fixing a great supper. Another surprise: she could cook with the expertise of a great line of Southern cooks. Then, if the day was a workday, I went to work at Fulton Drugstore until 11 p.m. When I came home, I found her ironing the clothes for the next day.

Although this sounds like a hard life, it did not seem so to us, because we were as one in our love, in our dedication to our small daughter, and in life. We were young, we were in love, and finally, we were together.

Ambition was a quality we both shared and understood. Four years of the hard scrabble of an enlisted man was not what I had in mind. I must make himself an officer. There were three ways to do so:

1. **Direct Commission: based on eight years of college, degrees, profession, etc. Needed political push in Washington.**

2. Medical School: upside—government would pay for it. Downside—had to pay back within eight years of service after graduation.

3. Officer Candidate School: the least desirable route. A very hard six months.

Nothing would ever be easy for us, so the O.C.S. came through first. Plans were made for her to return to Tampa for three months of underclass days. It was then that the first and perhaps the hardest blow hit the marriage.

In the midst of a frenzy of preparations to report to San Antonio for the spring session of O.C.S., Paula fell ill. This was unusual because she was ruggedly healthy. I took her to the doctor and was shocked to learn she was pregnant!

The shock was great, because as much as we both wanted a big family, now was not the time to get started.

"It never is," said Paula's mother who had had five children, each arriving at the wrong time.

We spent a horrible time discussing the problem, and always the answer was the same. An abortion. Both of us were against abortion, per se. However, we could not afford a child and go to O.C.S. and eventually on to medical school.

I knew the abortion mills of Juarez because I had served in an all-service medical inspection team, which kept an eye on the clinics. None of them could pass a test by U.S. standards, but one was close to acceptable. We chose that one. The fee was huge for us; it wiped out our savings. It was a considerable setback.

Then, too, just as Christmas, with all that extra spending, was coming on, we could not afford for Paula to miss work, and she would have to miss at least two weeks after the procedure.

The date was set. Christmas Eve. It couldn't be a worse date, but that was all that the clinic had available. After that they would close the door for two weeks for the holidays.

Traffic was bumper to bumper going over the bridge to Juarez. People decorated their cars for the holidays, horns were blowing, bands were playing, and everywhere people were having a great time.

In our 1951 Chevrolet we sat silently. Our daughter, Paula J., in a new wool dress with a hat, mittens, and an overcoat, looked adorable, and she was laughing and enjoying the crowd. Paula had on her stone face. When things got tough her face became rigid, hard to read. What could she be thinking? The last thing she thought she would ever endure as a happily married woman was an abortion. In our world, abortions were morally wrong and sinful and only resorted to by single girls or unhappily married wives, or for medical reasons. Not her. Not Paula, a happily married lady.

We could not find a spot to park, so we went round and round the block. The temperature was dropping. The car had no heater, and we were shivering.

The longer we procrastinated, the closer we came to calling it off. If she or I had said, "Forget it, let's go home," we would have lost our resolve.

Finally a parking spot in front of the clinic opened up. It was 6 p.m. We were on time.

The waiting room was dismal, but neat and clean. Paula J. played with knickknacks, entertaining herself as she always did. Paula maintained her icy calm, although she must have been boiling inside. I was a mess, because I, most of all, knew what could happen. This wasn't a U.S. hospital with surgical capabilities, anesthesiologists, and recuperative facilities. Many bad things could happen, with no way to fix them except prayers to God, and the end result was inevitable, *death!*

The doctor came out, addressed us pleasantly in Spanish, and shook my hand, and his face lit up in appreciation of Paula's beauty. Briefly, he said he had another case in front of us, but all in all, he wanted Paula J. and me to come back in two hours.

Two hours. An eternity. I took Paula J's little hand in mine and walked into the swirling happy holiday crowds.

I knew a very good restaurant, and because the maître d' knew me, I got a nice corner table overlooking the dance floor. It was a very good tourist trap, very family oriented, no rank floor show. All pure Mexican, a fine mariachi orchestra. Paula J. beamed at the music, and we ordered a nice supper.

I tried to stretch it out, but even with a floor show it was over in an hour. Still one more hour to go.

Out again mixing with the Christmas revelers, we went to the tourist shops, which had many toys to amuse Paula J., who was having a great time with me. Paula J. did not like it when people took up my time and attention and diverted attention from her time with her dad. This night she had me all to herself. We had had a great meal, had seen a mariachi band for the first time, and mingled with the crowds who were singing and dancing in the packed streets of sinful old Juarez. Christmas Eve. *Vaya.*

At 10 p.m. we went to the clinic again. Now, surely, she would be through. Pray God, she would be through. A grim-faced nurse cracked the door and said, in Spanish, that they had run into *un problemcito,* a little problem. There is no such thing as a little problem. I demanded to see the doctor, she said he was not there but had gone home to supper. It was *Noche buena,* she pointed out, the night Mexicans celebrate Christmas. I got hot and demanded his phone number. She refused and said to come back in two hours.

Two hours! Little Paula J. was already nuzzling into my shoulder, her little eyes flittering sleep but a moment away. I found my car, covered with parking tickets. I ripped them off the windshield angrily and threw them into the backseat. Fat chance I'd ever pay them.

The car was frigid. I tried to cover Paula J. with my coat, but nothing blunted that cold. I was praying so hard, I got an inspiration. Why not go to the main church and pray? Not only was it the appropriate place to pray, but it was a warm place to sit and meditate and let the two hours pass as Paula J. slept comfortably.

I sat in the front pew, Paula J. sprawled on the bench sleeping soundly, the exhausted sleep of a happy little girl with nothing on her mind but the toys she would get the next day when Santa would come and she would be happy.

I sat looking intently at the face of Jesus Christ on the cross. What a nerve I had to ask Him for help, on this night especially, on the night He was born! To come pray to Him when we were betraying all He taught to us. We were killing a child. A soul. We were committing the worse sin of all, murder.

There I sat filled with the anxieties of this world. The what-if world. What if we had the child? How to support it? How to go to O.C.S? What about medical school? All of the dreams of the future gone up in smoke. But, think again. What if she dies in that ratty clinic? What then? First of all, in the Air Force of that era I would be court-martialed and given a prison sentence. What would happen to Paula J? In one sudden moment she would lose both mother and father. Of course Paula's parents, the senator and his wife, would bring her up. But was it the same? Of course not. The enormity of my plight overcame me, and for the first time, since I was a baby, I cried. Cried unashamed tears. Of confusion, fright, guilt, a jumble of awful emotions. Suddenly a voice brought me back to Juarez.

"What are you doing here?" the voice sounded harsh and unfriendly. The priest shone a flashlight in his face.

"Praying," I said simply and truthfully. Isn't that what this church was for?

"You cannot be here. We are closed."

His voice was rough and gravelly.

I pointed to Christ on the cross.

"He is still here. I'm here to seek His help; I'm here to pray to Him. *Ayudame* [help me]. Surely you can leave us here alone. Let me stay one hour more."

"No. Get out or I'll call the police. If you want to pray come back tomorrow. We open at 6 a.m. It is Christmas. We have a big day tomorrow."

The priest seemed to soften a bit, as I picked up Paula J. I sensed the moment had come to beg. Perhaps the sight of the child in her father's arms would soften the priest.

"Please, Father. I'm in such need. Such turmoil. I'm losing my soul tonight. Might I pray with you? Confess to you? Help me, I ask you, as a lost soul."

"No," he said with finality. "You must go now; I must lock up the church and prepare it for Midnight Mass."

"I will also pray for your soul, for you may need it as much as I. You are a priest who has lost his calling."

I walked to the door, filled with rage and sadness. The priest seemed to be glad to see me depart. The heavy door clanged shut; I heard a lock turn.

What kind of a church is it that they must lock the doors, so the parishioners can't come in and pray to Jesus Christ? Surely, they are as wrong in their way as I was wrong in mine.

I took my time walking back to the clinic. I was cold again. I shivered and hugged Paula J. to me. She slept blissfully on, no part of the dilemma that engulfed her parents.

It was 11:45 p.m. when I banged on the doctor's door. Now I was determined to kick the door down if necessary. Surely she needed a transfusion. Did they have blood, the right type and cross match? To Mexican doctors of that day, blood was blood. Red was red. There was no difference.

"I told you at midnight," her voice was softer now. "She is okay, out of danger. Let her rest until midnight; then you take her."

All of the rage and turmoil disappeared. She is well. She is alive. She'll live. Nothing wrong. I crumpled into a big easy chair and Paula J. awoke for a moment, hugged my neck and went back to sleep.

It was one of the finest Christmases we ever spent in all the short time we were married. Paula had had a painful time. She needed several transfusions, but she was a very strong Southern woman. She was a survivor. In one week she was back to work, looking sleek and beautiful. And so another major hurdle was passed. It brought us much closer together. Daily, I prayed thanking God for His mercy, but really, I have never gotten over doing that apparently necessary thing. Murder is murder, and unforgivable. Period.

O.C.S. was every bit as hard and stupid as I had envisioned, relieved only by the pink envelopes that arrived from home. The second three months was a day at the beach. She came, with the child, and found a nice apartment, and we enjoyed a more ample salary and the collegiate atmosphere of the training.

Again, fate dealt a curveball. The Korean War was almost finished, and the Air Force did not need 615 new officers. We were given a choice, which in my case proved to be to serve out the remaining six months on my two-year requirement at the grade of staff sergeant in the pharmacy at the old base in El Paso.

But fate intervened. Angered because I had not gotten a response from the University of Miami medical school, I wired them. I would soon be discharged. What to do filled my thoughts. Certainly not return to La Economica in Ybor City and work as a druggist. I began to worry about what to do in Tampa, when suddenly all was solved.

The medical school informed me that I was accepted, and suddenly my lifelong dream of becoming a doctor was within my grasp. Excitedly I informed Paula, and true to her combative, ambitious spirit, she agreed to accept it. Life as a doctor with her was life as I envisioned it.

Miami was heaven after El Paso. She came and set up an attractive apartment in Coral Gables and then went home. The first semester of medical school was a 24-hour-a-day grind. Once again I waited for the pink envelopes, only now I missed the child as well, because she had become very important to me. She was cute, intelligent, and as much fun as her mother.

When I started the second semester, tragedy struck home.

Death of a Hero

As usual, I had a terrible New Year's Eve in 1955. At the time I was married to my first wife, Paula, who was absolutely wonderful. But that particular New Year's Eve, I tossed and turned in bed at my in-laws' house. I was in my first year of medical school and had the important mid-year exams on my mind, and so going to a society party was a waste of precious time. Moreover, I had a black presentiment of something bad hanging over me.

The phone rang at 5 a.m. I knew that that call would not be good.

"Are you Ferdie Pacheco? Do you have a father named J.B. Pacheco?"

"Yes. What's the matter?"

"We've been trying to locate his relatives. He's had a heart attack; he's at the Centro Asturiano Hospital."

"I'll be there!"

I jumped in my car and sped down Bayshore Boulevard toward the hospital, with my heart sinking. There, in a freezing corridor, lined up with other gurneys, was my father. No one had recognized him, in spite of the fact that he was almost famous and the owner of La Economica Drugstore, a few blocks from the hospital.

The intern on duty on New Year's Eve had just arrived from Cuba and didn't know a soul in the Ybor City. He'd given Papa some Demerol and stacked him in the corridor. It was criminal negligence.

Immediately, I whisked him to Trelles Clinic, called a cardiologist, and started treatment. Precious hours had passed, and with them the chances of recovery grew dimmer.

His eyes fluttered awake. He smiled when he saw me sitting by his side holding his hand.

"Don't worry, I'm here. I love you, Pop."

At least I got to say that.

"I won't let anything happen to you."

He smiled and gripped my hand hard.

"When you get out of here, we'll sell the drugstore. Then, when I'm a doctor, I'll take care of you and mom for the rest of your life. Your worries are over!"

I tried to sound optimistic. He moved his massive head so that he could whisper into my ear, "Just do for your kids what I did for you."

I'd heard him say that many times. Still, I was going to take care of him until the end.

We held hands until he went limp. By 6 a.m. he was gone. J.B. Pacheco, my powerhouse of a father, was gone. At least he got to see me get into medical school, if not graduate as a doctor. Had that stupid prank not cost me five years, my father would have lived to see me graduate as a doctor.

The Lord indeed works in mysterious ways. He let me go, forgave me, and made me pay a hard price as punishment.

Tragic Love Reprise

Now, with the GI Bill paying the tuition and a third of the sale of La Economica Drugstore, it became a dim possibility to pay my way through school. Of course, Miami was not El Paso. Prices doubled and tripled, and as the baby grew to school age, and educational expenses were added, and soon, we faced economic ruin again. Again Paula took control, swung a good job with Haynes Hose, and we only needed my work as a pharmacist on weekends to make it. Again, the cycle of hard work, isolation, and accomplishment repeated itself.

When people are buried in the day-to-day struggle to survive, they do not notice the slow erosion of their interpersonal relationships. A love as strong and hot as ours is presumed to outlast anything. But a love relationship is fragile. Few are ironclad. Few people are lucky enough to commit to each other for life, no matter what.

The sad day came when it became apparent that we were in a corner. Years were flying by. Her good years. She was even more beautiful than before. Her father was now a state senator and needed her in Tallahassee. I hated the thought of depriving her of that wonderful opportunity to work with her father. With her looks and the free and loose life in the state capital, it appeared that I could not permit her to place herself in that position. Years of medical education remained ahead. There was no shortcut. My pride would not allow thoughts of a loan from my family or hers. We had gotten this far together, as a team, and we were so close. So very close.

But, it was not meant to be, and so, on a bright, sunny Miami day she drove up with her mother, took a very few personal things, and left.

"Just ask her to stay," whispered my mother-in-law.

"I can't. It has to come from her."

It didn't.

My world had come to an end. I missed her terribly. I missed the child almost as much. Once, we were the perfect family. Once, we were the best bet for success. She was beloved by my classmates and their wives. I was envied. Now she was gone.

Did we still love one another? Yes, in our own way. The problem had no answer. I had not come this close to graduation to quit now. Nor would she have wanted me to.

We had been through much. We grew up together, because I had been as immature and innocent of life as she, and together we had faced life and learned, matured, grown up. One part of each was carried by the other. Whatever future life had in store for us we would always look at it, and part of our subconscious mind would say, "I wonder what he/she would think of this new achievement." She would go on with life, her enormous beauty now augmented by her talent, her intelligence, and her individuality. She became a unique individual, a great woman, ruggedly going her own way, even when wrong, and somehow, winning in the game of life. She did well, marrying a senator and raising a family. Somehow I felt some impact on her life, some responsibility for her success. I did well, acknowledging quietly that some part of my success was due to her and her support in the hard times. What we had not been able to accomplish together, we accomplished apart.

CHAPTER 4

From the Ghetto to Ali

After I got my medical degree from the University of Miami and completed my internship at Mount Sinai Hospital as a physician, in June 1959, I headed for Miami's black ghetto, Overtown, to fulfill my father's dream for me—to help the indigent.

Overtown was tough and tragic, but I was desperately needed by its 20,000 poor blacks, who were segregated from Miami's white community—and its doctors. I announced my fees: five dollars for an office visit, if you could pay it; if not, you could charge it; no pediatric fees for babies I delivered until they were two years old; and no charge for old-timers 60 years and up.

I saw 50 to 100 people a day and had the greatest nurse, Mabel Norwood, who stayed with me for 25 years. Our office was open from 9 a.m. until 8 p.m., and I worked like a dog. Boy, was I cool in that neighborhood! They treated me like kin, and I loved every minute of it.

A few months later, when the Cuban refugees came to Miami following Fidel Castro's revolution, I opened a second office to serve them. Same deal with fees, but the Cubans didn't need much help, because they had white skin and played on a different field.

My second office was referred to as the *white office*. Liberals today breathe hard when I speak of a *black office* or a *white office*, but that's the way it was back then in the days of segregation in the South. The fact that I had these two separate but very equal offices opened the door to my life in boxing.

Working in the Overtown ghetto was the culmination of all I had studied for when my father told me I had to help the poor. But I hadn't anticipated the all-encompassing poverty of the ghetto, and its endless tragedies and sadness. I had grown up in a loving family in a nurturing community, and I was upbeat and happy by nature. Now hip-deep in daily tragedy, I needed something to lighten my load and forget the pain, a distraction. Miraculously, the recollection of a cherished childhood memory came to me one day and led me to rediscovering an old love that would save me.

I was eight years old, playing in a baseball game, and the score was about 50-45. Around the 28th inning, my mother called me to come running. I quickly bathed and dressed in my Sunday best. My father was coming to take me to the Columbia Restaurant, the best restaurant in Florida.

The Columbia? For lunch? At 2 p.m.? But at eight years old, I asked no questions when my father showed up. I knew it was something big because he wore a tie.

When we got to the Columbia, we were ushered onto the patio, which was empty except for a single table where two men sat. I recognized one, the owner, Lawrence Hernandez, who rose to greet us with a big hug. The other man sat in front of a steaming plate of *Arroz con Pollo* (chicken with yellow rice). He was huge, and his face fit the description "ruggedly handsome."

Lawrence said, "This is Jack Dempsey, the heavyweight champion of the world."

I'd never seen someone so big, but I bravely thrust out my hand, looked him in the eye (as I had been taught by Papa), and said, "Please to meetcha, Mr. Champ. I'm Ferdie Pacheco."

His huge hand swallowed mine.

"Had lunch yet?" he asked in a kindly voice.

I had, but I sensed that he wanted me to keep him company while he ate, so I said, "No, sir."

In a flash, he scooped me up, sat me on his lap, and handed me a fork.

"Dig in," he said. "I like little boys that kin eat."

What an experience! Between bites, Dempsey told one amazing boxing story after another. When he was through, he placed me down in front of him.

"You know anything about boxing?" he asked.

"I read my friend's brother's *Ring* magazines," I said.

We loved boxing and sparred all of the time on our block.

"So you know about me?" he asked.

"I know about The Long Count," I said, referring to Dempsey's infamous bout with Gene Tunney.

"Ouch. Let's change the subject," said Dempsey, getting a big laugh from the men. "Show me your guard."

I stood, left foot out, left hand extended, ready to jab with my right up against my face, which was tucked behind my left shoulder.

"You know what a one-two punch is?" the Champ asked.

I did, but I knew he wanted to show me, so I said I didn't.

"First the left jab, which you might block," he said, and gently lifted his gigantic left fist against my forehead. "And then comes the right hand."

I relaxed as he faked hitting me with his right, then, zoom! A quick left hook bounced off my jaw.

I knew he was holding back, but I could still feel a hint of the jolt.

"That's the part of the one-two that knocks 'em out. The left hook is the killer," Dempsey said.

"But you said you'd show me the one-two. That wasn't a real one-two, Champ," I said, feeling that he'd cheated to make me the butt of a joke.

The men laughed appreciatively.

"Protect yourself at all times," he said, in a hard, guttural voice, and then grabbed me and gave me a hug. "At all times."

Soon, it was time to go. But first we split a bowl of *flan* (Cuban egg custard), he lit up a *Puro* (a Cuban cigar) sipped a demitasse of black Cuban coffee, and then made me stand in front of him. He looked me in the eye.

"So you won't forget me, Champ, I'm giving you these gloves. Will you remember me by them?"

He handed me a tiny pair of inscribed golden boxing gloves to put on my keychain. One glove had "J" and the other "D." They sat on the bottom of a tiny cardboard box, resting on a little square of white cotton. Tears welled up in my eyes, but I quickly jumped for his neck before he noticed. I didn't want the grownups to see me cry and embarrass my father.

I had those boxing gloves on my keychain through 12 years of college, through the Air Force in the Korean War, and my internship at Mt. Sinai Hospital in Miami Beach.

My memory of Dempsey and my love of boxing helped me to find something to distract me from my daily grind in Overtown—and begin the next phases of my life.

The Doctor in the Gym

By 1960, I was a regular at Miami Beach promoter Chris Dundee's Tuesday Night Fights.

Boy, were they great. Chris was a top boxing promoter. He genuinely loved boxing. I sat ringside, in the corner where his brother, the great cornerman-trainer-manager, Angelo Dundee worked. Angelo was at the beginning of his long distinguished career and had yet to win a championship.

The Dundees had a major problem. They had no doctor's facilities to which to send their injured black boxers. In those days of segregation, they were accepted only in the ghetto.

The door of opportunity opened, and I was there, well prepared to step through it. I already had a black office (and a white office for the rest).

To illustrate the absurdity of racism and segregation, the Cuban boxers were all black except for Luis Manuel Rodriquez, Sugar Ramos, Mantequilla Napoles, Baby Luis, Robinson Garcia, and Douglas Vallant—they all insisted on coming to the white office.

"We're not black; we're Cuban," they said. And in Cuban Miami, they were. Amazing!

So I became the doctor for the Fifth Street Gym and treated all of the fighters who passed through there for the next 20 years. I made a deal with Chris that he couldn't refuse: free medical care for the boxers and their retinues, which ultimately included all of their families, too.

I treated Muhammad Ali for 17 years and took no fees. I paid for everything: X-rays, lab work, consultations, and physical therapy. Everything.

Chris Dundee repaid me in coin of the realm; he welcomed me into the deepest insides of boxing. Let me tell you, boxing gets deep. I worked the corners, accompanied fighters to Rome and London, and became as trusted as you could get. I became "a boxing guy," one of "us." It was a big title, one I was very proud of, because it meant that I was accepted.

To illustrate this point, Bob Foster, the light heavyweight champion of the world, once came to Miami to fight Vincent Rondon, a fighter I worked with at the gym. But Foster had a bad case of the flu. He needed a shot. Chris called me; I came to the gym during my lunch to treat Foster. Horrified, he balked.

"Hey, he works for Rondon," Foster said, refusing the shot. "He ain't gonna shoot me."

"In here [the Fifth Street Gym], he works for no one," admonished Foster's tough manager, Lou Vizcusi. "He's a Fight Doc! He's one of us."

That was it. Foster took the shot and knocked out my guy within 30 seconds of the first round. Some shot!

Corner Work

Working a boxing corner may seem like it ought to be exciting and a lot of fun. Well, it's about as much fun as cutting grass. It's a routine—easy to do and bereft of fun. It's repetitive scut work and a drag.

Let me amend that. It is a lot of fun if the fight is a toe-to-toe war, a matchup of championship significance. For example, if you're working Muhammad Ali versus Joe Frazier in the "Thrilla in Manila" at noon on a sweltering hot midday, and the fight has reached life-and-death proportions, well, hell yes, it is the most excitement you can handle in life—short of combat in a real war.

But in more than 20 years of working fights, there are a few dozen of that kind and thousands of pure boredom.

Three men work a corner, although a boxer actually only needs the chief cornerman, normally. When the bell rings at the end of a round, the stool man brings the stool in the ring and places it when the boxer reaches the corner. The second man splashes cold water on the boxer's face and head to refresh him, and then wipes it off. All three men search for damage.

Some corners have cut-men, who have their *stuff* with them to stop a cut, but strict regulations have limited the stuff to adrenaline. Totally outlawed is the old *dynamite,* a corrosive solution of ferrous sulfate, which would char the tissue and stop bleeding. It was highly dangerous to the eye and could blind a boxer. When the fight finished the *cut man* had to cut out all of the burned tissue or else it would stay in place as a big lump of scar tissue, which would reopen all the time. Thank goodness that evil is gone.

Only one man speaks in a top professional corner. I was lucky enough to observe the magic of Angelo Dundee, who was the chief cornerman. He ordered us to work on various things. Luis Sarria, the physical conditioner, massaged the boxer's tired arms and legs to get the blood working again. As The Fight Doctor, I took care of the rest of the small injuries. While we worked, Angelo talked. The fighter had to be able to hear Angelo, because Angelo was giving him round-to-round battle instructions. A genius like Angelo can win a fight through his instructions or by the use of psychology. He has to be inside the fighter's head. And a fighter has to execute his orders.

A cornerman must invent new ways to wake up a fighter, to get his mind back on the battle. I tried anything.

One night, a wonderful young Cuban fighter, Frank Otero, was going to sleep on me. So as we stood in the corner waiting for the bell to ring, I took the top of the ice bag off and poured the contents, ice cubes and ice water, into his big protector.

Frankie's eyes opened wide, and he let out a yell.

Then he said, in a surprisingly calm voice, "Doc, was that absolute necessary?"

All of the teamwork in a corner must happen in 60 seconds and then the cornermen must get out of the ring or be disqualified. Sounds easy? It is if you have a team who has worked together for years. The best corner I ever worked was with Angelo and Sarria.

There's a great sense of accomplishment, a rush of emotion, and elation when you win, whether it's a world championship or a 10-round preliminary fight with a young fighter just starting. There aren't many moments like that in life. It makes up for the thousands of *dog* nights, which are boring.

But I never regretted a minute. It was my ticket into the topsy-turvy world of boxing.

Angelo and I formed a team. I'd go all over the world with him, watch him work his magic, and develop 12 champions, and as the cherry on the cake, he brought Cassius Clay, a kid, to my little office on N.W. Second Avenue and 10th Street.

Clay was tall, beautifully sculpted, and handsome of face. And a nonstop talking machine. When he left my office after the first visit, my wise nurse, Miss Mabel, shook her head and said, "My, my. Either that boy is crazy as a loon, or he is going to be the Heavyweight Champion of the World."

How right she was.

CHAPTER 5

Ali: An Evaluation After 30 Years

After hundreds of interviews, TV specials, three books, and two movies, I am still in awe of the fact that I was a part of Muhammad Ali's life.

Ali surely is one of the best-known people of our age. His fame is worldwide and all encompassing, not just restricted to the field of sports or even the boundaries of the United States.

Interviewers still troop through my study. They set up their cameras, consult their notes, and ask the same questions over and over, but my patience has long since run out. Those who start with the question, "How did you meet Muhammad Ali?" are thrown out of my house immediately. They aren't serious and haven't done their homework. I've written three books on Ali. Everything has been said. Read them before you come over!

But when I sat down to write this book, I realized I had to analyze the Ali phenomenon. Who was he? Why was he so universally accepted? What kind of intelligence did he have? Why was he so sexy? Who exactly is Muhammad Ali?

In good conscience, I cannot skip my relations with him. I can't ignore him. I also cannot overlook the fact that he made me almost famous.

Almost famous is what I have been during the 40 years I spent in boxing, riding in the Ali circus, and the years following in televised sports. I have Ali to thank. As he says to all of us at every Ali circus reunion, "I made you all famous!"

A German publisher called and wanted 4,000 words on why Ali is sexy. I laughed and said, "I don't need 4,000 words. I need four. 'Just look at him!'"

It is the first thing that strikes you. Ali has an exceptional physiognomy. His proportions are perfect. His face is innocent in its handsomeness. His skin is smooth, with a light, attractive tan shade, a quality inherited from his mom, Odessa. He is an eternally beautiful man-child.

At first, he seems shorter than six foot four, his actual height. Because of his baby face and open, funny way, boxers never saw his size until they faced him in the ring. They'd invariably say in a shocked voice, "But he's so big." By then, it was too late.

Sonny Liston was one of the best examples of this. He was shocked when they faced off in 1964. Accustomed to being the big guy, the intimidator, Liston found himself looking up to Ali.

✗✗✗✗✗✗✗

To address the greatest misconception about Ali: Is he intelligent, as in very smart? Is he a thinking person?

No, Ali is not an intelligent man, at least not in the conventional sense. He's been famous since he was 17. Reading did not come easily to him, so he does not bother with newspapers, magazines, or books. His taste in movies remains at an infantile level with B-horror movies and awful cowboy films. He barely got through high school and could not pass the most basic Army intelligence test.

Almost every conversation centered on him. If authors like Budd Schulberg or Norman Mailer came to see him, would Ali be interested in what they had done in their lives and in their writing? No. Ali spoke about Ali. Period. Nothing else interested him. He was an expert on Ali. No need to ask him about anything else.

What Ali did have was an amazing ability to instinctively do the right thing. It had nothing to do with an intellectual thought process. He was intuitive. He "felt" things. He was flighty, which is why the Honorable Elijah Muhammad told his son Herbert, Ali's manager, "Make sure you are the last face he sees and the last voice he hears before he goes to bed."

In boxing, Ali did everything differently from anyone in the gym. And almost all of it was wrong.

The gray old men of the Fifth Street Gym shook their heads as they watched the sleek young dancer glide around the ring, jabbing and dropping his hands to his side. They would shift their dead cigar butts to the side of the mouth and say, "If he drops his left after a jab, a good boxer will cross him with a straight right and kill the kid."

They all nodded in agreement, and then, with mouths agape, they would see Ali pull his head back from a punch.

"*That* would get him *moidered* in the big leagues," they'd say. "You pull your head back, and then what? Where are you going to go when you've gone back as far as you can? The next shot catches you all stretched out and starches you. He'd better change that!"

Then they would watch in amazement as Ali worked out with top contenders and champions (Ingemar Johansson once worked with him and dismissed him after two rounds because he couldn't hit Ali at *all*).

No one could connect solidly with the young kid. Why? Because he was a meteor. His reflexes were razor sharp, and his size gave him a huge advantage. Ali made mistakes, but when a fighter tried to capitalize on them, he missed but got a lot of Ali leather in his face for his efforts.

Wise, old Eddie Futch, the legendary cornerman who managed and trained the fierce Joe Frazier, put it best, "Ali showed you his mistakes, and when you fell in his trap to take advantage, he killed you."

✗✗✗✗✗✗✗

As great a boxer as Ali was, it was a distinct surprise that he was not good at, nor cared about, other athletic endeavors. He couldn't swim; dance; play football, basketball or baseball; shoot pool; play golf or tennis, and he didn't care to try.

This sort of typifies genius, I suppose. People who are the best in their field are rarely good at other things. They practice their craft to the exclusion of all else. Thus Picasso only did art, Rubinstein the piano, Isaac Stern the violin. Maybe that's what it takes to be the best in the world.

✗✗✗✗✗✗✗

What about Ali's sensuality, his sex appeal, his hypnotic appeal to women? Why was he so special?

Power, of course; the ultimate aphrodisiac, and the celebrity that goes with it. Ali was the most recognized man in the world.

After Ali's bewildering victory in Zaire in 1974—where he once again used his intuition, ignoring the advice of his corner, and invented the rope-a-dope, correctly guessing it would exhaust George

Foreman and result in a knockout—I rode back to our base camp at N'Zelle with boxing historian and author Budd Schulberg, a shrewd observer of the heavyweight scene.

A veritable monsoon splattered us and obscured our vision; off to the side, we detected some movement, but in the dark of the jungle we could not make it out. Then, as dawn broke and the first rays of the sun lit the dark jungle, we discovered what that movement had been.

Groups of natives had gathered at the roadside to watch us pass. They lined both sides of the highway. Women held up their babies so they could see the great champion, Muhammad Ali, as he drove by. They could say they had seen a great warrior pass. As the rain fell harder, they stayed, holding corrugated sheets of tin or palm fronds over the babies' heads.

We watched in silence from the darkness of the bus, and I said to Schulberg, "We are watching the transformation of Ali from champion of the United States to champion of the world."

And so it was. No matter where we went—an obscure village in India, a settlement in the Gaza, anywhere—people got the eight-by-10 glossies, pamphlets, and posters. Everyone seemed to own an Ali T-shirt. The world was his, though he remained a simple, uncomplicated, and happy man.

This quality, his happiness with himself, made him reach out to everyone. He wanted them to love him as he loved himself. He seemed to be saying, "Look at how good [how pretty, how funny] I am. You want to hear a poem? See my magic tricks? Here I am. Love me; come get a piece of this." And he seduced the world! Oscar Wilde once said, "To love oneself is the beginning of a lifelong romance." When Ali does the self-love bit, it's hard as hell not to agree with the champ. He is impossible not to love.

Ali was the most available superstar ever. He reveled in being with his fans or surprising the unwary with a sudden appearance.

One nasty winter afternoon in Cleveland, Ali peered out his limo's window and saw a group of working women, tired after their nine-hour factory shifts, patiently waiting for the bus to take them home to prepare supper and continue their lives of quiet desperation.

Ali stopped the limo and hopped out. With no bodyguards or flunkies, he grabbed one astonished woman, gave her a big bear hug, kissed her on the mouth, and jived with her.

"Ooh Mama, what kind of man you married to that lets you out here in the street all alone? You so fine, I may come by here some afternoon and snatch you away!"

The women screamed in delight and ecstasy. He didn't stop until he showered attention on each one, then he hopped back into his limo, and rode off.

This insistence that every person fall in love with Ali is what made him so lovable. I never found anyone who could resist him.

✗✗✗✗✗✗

Ali had great instincts and dealt with his problems intuitively. Many times his decisions seemed wildly at odds with what logic would dictate. The biggest one was his decision to refuse induction into the Army in 1967. Much of the country turned against him and called him a traitor—or worse. He was a villain, roundly detested.

But three years later, he was America's hero again. History proved Ali right; the war in Vietnam was wrong.

I offer this as a prime example of Ali intuitively choosing the right way in spite of opposing viewpoints.

In my opinion, Ali couldn't have passed the Army intelligence test that he would've had to take when he was drafted and refused induction. With a bit of Don King trickeration, some racial flak by the Muslims, and high-priced legal footwork, I'm sure that Ali would have ultimately been turned down by the Army. And if inducted, he would have just done a two-year stint like Joe Louis or Elvis Presley.

But it was the Muslims who saw value in stirring up the nation's racial wars by having Ali thrown out of boxing. Yet when Ali refused induction, it was the Muslims who betrayed him. They realized they had cut the golden goose's neck and were now expected to support him.

The Honorable Elijah Muhammad, trying to cut his losses, threw Ali out of the Muslims, forbade him from using his Muslim name, barred him from his mosques, and even denied him the right to speak to fellow Muslims. The last proscription was patently stupid because Ali's manager was Elijah's wastrel son, Herbert. At the first hint of a prospective fight, that restriction was quickly lifted.

Poor Ali. He had a wife, a growing family, and no way to make a living. We all pitched in. A pal of mine, producer Zef Bufman, put Ali in a dismal Broadway musical that opened and closed in seven days. But Ali still got paid. Then Murray Warner, a radio and TV producer, invented computer-simulated boxing. He hit on the idea of having an undefeated Ali face an undefeated Rocky Marciano.

We turned the computer simulation into a script, secured a gym with Angelo Dundee, got his brother Chris to referee, and I acted as a corner man. We had huge fun.

We filmed 15 different endings. The decision we showed depended on where you viewed the fight. In New York and Chicago, Ali won; in Philly (with its big Italian and black audience) it was a draw. In Italy, Marciano knocked out Ali—who made a tidy sum from all of these virtual matches.

But it wasn't enough.

Then Ali's luck kicked in. He was booked on a speaking tour of predominantly white colleges, and a few black ones, too. It was a shock to everyone (except Ali) that the white kids loved him.

Slowly, public opinion began to turn. The college kids agreed with Ali's position on Vietnam. From all over the country (and Canada), they followed Ali's tour.

By the time of his first bout with Frazier in 1971, Ali had a huge white fan base of college kids. He had become America's folk hero and has never relinquished that position. White or black, Muhammad Ali is the man, our man.

It was safe to love Ali. When he shouted from the rooftops that he was totally uninterested in white women, he neutered the racial monster. He made it abundantly clear that he was not attracted to white women.

One time, as we exited from our hotel elevator and pushed our way through a lobby crowded with fans, Ali came face to face with one of the most beautiful (white) women I'd ever seen. She tenderly grasped his hand, pressing her room key into it, along with an unspoken invitation. Ali looked at the key as if it were a coiled mamba snake. He let it fall on the marble floor, where it clattered embarrassingly loud. The woman walked on, and Ali rushed to the exit as quickly as he could.

To the public at large, no other black athlete or entertainer was so appealing, yet so safe. Who could not love Ali, the married man with children and fervent religious beliefs, who was obviously comfortable in his own skin?

Who could resist Ali? No one.

✗✗✗✗✗✗

Among Ali's most endearing qualities is his spontaneous generosity to strangers.

Returning from Zaire after the "Rumble in the Jungle," I was seated next to an elderly gentleman in first class. Angelo Dundee had just finished reading the newspapers' coverage of the bout, and he'd brought them for me to read. The older fellow read along with me over my shoulder.

"Do you have anything to do with Mister Ali?" the old gentleman asked, as he sipped his sherry.

"Yes, I am his doctor," I said, expecting to hear an Ali story from this distinguished-looking man. I wasn't disappointed.

"My grandson graduated from MIT this spring. I gave him his graduation present, a three-month Euro Rail pass, plus a small stipend so he could stay in youth hostels throughout Europe. The only stipulation I made was that he had to be back in America in time to begin his first job in Atlanta, Georgia."

I couldn't guess what this had to do with Ali, but the old man, who had flown with the Lafayette Escadrille in World War I, was taking his time spinning the yarn and enjoying it.

He explained that the boy was almost late. He had landed at Kennedy Airport and hustled out to the expressway to hitchhike to Atlanta. It was late in the afternoon, drizzly, and unseasonably cold. He looked like a hippie with long hair, scraggly beard, and rumpled clothes. His chances of getting picked up were slim.

Suddenly a black Rolls Royce pulled up. In the backseat sat the heavyweight champion, Muhammad Ali, smiling at him quizzically.

"Where do you think you're going in weather like this? Who you think's gonna pick you up looking like Charles Manson?" Ali laughed.

Ali's charm put the boy at ease. In a flood of words he told the champ of his trouble. He had to get to Atlanta or he'd lose his first job. But worse, he'd break his word and his grandfather's heart.

Without asking the boy, Ali took him to his home in Cherry Hill, New Jersey. His wife prepared a sumptuous feast. Then Ali gave him a choice. What movies would he like to see? Old Ali fights? Monster-horror films? Old cowboy movies from the 1950s?

Of course, the boy picked the fight films, and Ali narrated them in his inimitable style, shouting and laughing. After the show, the boy was sent to the guest bedroom to sleep.

Next morning, he awoke to the aroma of breakfast, which Ali was in the kitchen fixing. It was just after dawn, and Ali's wife was still asleep.

After breakfast, the boy and Ali got into the Rolls and drove to the expressway. Except, to the boy's surprise, they went straight to the airport.

The big car stopped, and Ali handed the boy a ticket to Atlanta.

"Here, you'll get there in time now," he said.

"I can't pay you. I'm broke," the surprised boy said.

"Yes, you can. When you get going in your first job, you'll send me the money."

"That's a promise," the boy said.

"And if you can't afford it, that's all right, too," said Ali, giving the boy a quick hug and pat on the shoulder.

Sitting next to me on the plane, the old man's eyes glistened.

"No wonder they call him champion. Ali personifies the word," he said.

Generosity, kindness, and a strong desire to help are the factors that make Ali attractive to people all over the world.

Thrilla in Manila

Ali's ability to make his opponents feel safe was most evident in the third fight with Frazier on October 1, 1975, in Manila. This was a brutal, primitive contest of flesh, blood, and will. Ali came back to his corner after the 10th round and said, "This is the closest I've come to dying."

He was dehydrated, exhausted by the brutal pace, hurt by Frazier's thunderous punches, and bewildered by his willingness to take awful punishment and inflict some of his own.

The fight, which Ali won on a technical knockout in the 14th round, was so close to life and death that it finally made me reevaluate my own role as a doctor in the fighter's corner.

Did I need to be part of this brutality? Should I even be in a corner? Corner work is exactly the opposite of doctor work. Somehow you're drawn into the mystique, the fun, the drama, and, yes, the spotlight shining on you as one of the four men who worked in Ali's corner. I had been able to ignore that nagging question of conscience: Could I justify being there? Looking at two men risking their lives, the answer ultimately was no. Nothing was worth this.

But I stayed on after that epic battle out of loyalty to Ali, though I knew that The Champ was falling apart. I knew that "The Thrilla in Manila" was the last stop on the road to boxing damage.

After a grim battle, each subsequent match caused Ali more brain and kidney damage. What happened was progressive, irreversible, and, regrettably, inevitable.

It is a little-known fact that the Manila fight was stopped by kind Eddie Futch for a reason, not obvious to the press, the fans, or Ali's corner. We were too relieved to see it end to wonder about the why of it.

Futch lived to a ripe old age and was a walking encyclopedia of boxing history dating back to Joe Louis's day. He said to me when we did a TV special for Showtime called *The 12 Greatest Rounds of Boxing,* "Frazier was legally blind in his right eye. How he passed the vision test, only promoter Don King knows, but, hey, it's Manila, and we had a much-awaited fight on tap." Eddie clearly regretted but also accepted how things were—had to be—in the fight biz.

Let me say right here, unequivocally, that none of us in Ali's camp knew about Frazier's eye problems. What an advantage that would have given us! If we knew that he had only one good eye, we would have worked exclusively on that eye and soon Frazier would have been blind. But we didn't know. Had we known, I would have had a curious dilemma. As a doctor and an advocate for boxing safety, it would have been my duty to stop the fight before it took place. People would have stood in line to take a shot at me, starting with Philippines president Ferdinand Marcos, promoter Don King, Herbert, and his avaricious dad, the Honorable Elijah Muhammad, and the boxing world in general.

But the best fight in heavyweight history took place as scheduled before a sellout crowd in Manila on a sweltering, humid morning. (Yes, morning, so the fight would play live in arenas and theaters all over the United States in the evening.)

As the 13th and 14th rounds escalated in fury and intensity, Ali set his traps. Frazier stumbled into each one. All along, Ali hit hard rights, which began closing Frazier's left eye (his good one!).

That ended the war of attrition. Frazier's left eye closed, and as we now know, he was legally blind in his right eye. Could Futch send a totally sightless Frazier to face the hard-punching Ali, who was determined to knock his fighter out once and for all?

No.

That fight, above all, established a high watermark for Ali's courage, tenacity, and willingness to accept brutal punishment, and it defined his determination to win and inability to admit defeat. I guess, all things considered, that fight defined the word *champion.*

So Ali, with his baby face and joking way of looking at life, was tougher than the rest. Inside the ring, Ali was the toughest man on the planet! But then Father Time arrived, and things changed.

Why I Quit Ali

I had a long time to think on my way home from Manila. I said to my wife Luisita, "I gotta get out!" I thought maybe if I quit and made a statement and the press picked it up, Ali would quit of his own accord.

Fat chance! The last one to realize what is happening to himself is the boxer. Behind him is an army of bloodsuckers who make a handsome living hanging onto their places on the caboose. This army is not restricted to a few poor ghetto bums. I'm talking about the head of a religious order, the owner of Vegas casinos, the heads of TV networks, the media, and on down to the poorest boxing scribe, and greedy bloodsucker promoters.

I knew I would lose, be reviled, and called a traitor, etc. Yes, yes, all of that, but Ali listened and said, "Well, he's right." Ali and I have never exchanged a cross word. Most of the crowd that reviled me in the worst terms, now come up to me and whisper, "You was right, Doc."

Jumping off the Ali circus express was one of the hardest things I ever did in all my years in boxing. First of all, I loved the guy and I loved being part of history. I loved working in the corner in the Rumble in the Jungle, the Liston fights, and the greatest fight I ever saw, the Thrilla in Manila. That was very special to me. Being part of the Ali entourage opened doors to me in Hollywood and New York. His was a gigantic sun, illuminating the world of sports. All else, including loud-mouth broadcaster Howard Cosell, diminished in his presence and couldn't even cast a shadow.

But as all humans must, Ali grew old. The first thing that goes is the reflexes. Ali had the fastest in boxing history. That's why he never got hit. With the reflexes slowed, everybody hit Ali. The beating he took in Manila from Joe Frazier almost cost him his life. It finished whatever little he had left in his brain. His brain was a swollen, scar-filled mess. Anyone with eyes could see the difference in his speech, now slurred and slowing—in slowing of ideation, the lack of balance, the shuffling gait, and the loss of reflexes. As a doctor, I couldn't in all consciousness stay knowing what I knew. There was little I could do but to tell him to quit.

Of all of those who should have stepped off the Ali circus express with me, the only one who couldn't make himself do it was Angelo Dundee.

I am very close to Angelo, and I am grateful for his dragging me with him to hundreds of great fights. He is a generous, kind, softhearted man.

Angelo had one fault: He loved greatness in a boxer, and in Ali, he had had the best. How could he leave now, when Ali needed him the most?

I understood and said nothing in the press.

Angelo had his mantra: "I was with him when he started, and I want to be there when he finishes."

Then as if in a second afterthought, he offered this rationalization, "I'm in the corner to protect him. If he is taking a beating and I can protect him, I'll stop the fight."

Yes, but he didn't.

Because Angelo never had that choice. Only Herbert and the Muslims had that option. Not Angelo.

When Ali fought Ken Norton in San Diego in 1973, Ken broke Ali's jaw in the first round. He had 11 more to go. The jaw was fractured straight through. Very dangerous. I said to stop it right there. Angelo agreed, but Ali said, "No!" Herbert and the Muslims said, "No!" How would it look, Ali, the greatest black athlete in the world, quitting on a stool? The fight went on.

"Uh, oh," I thought, "nothing short of death can stop an Ali fight."

Frazier came close in Manila. Larry Holmes came close in Vegas five years later. Where was Angelo then? Angelo was a cog in the wheel. The wheel was Herbert, Ali, and the Muslims.

Finally, a New York Boxing Authority doctor showed me disastrous lab results. Ali's kidneys were falling apart. He would not be allowed to fight in New York! That's it, bub, I'm outta here. I stayed too long. Most of the damage you see today could have been avoided if he had quit after Manila.

Even his training was highly destructive. As his three sparring partners, he had three future champions, Larry Holmes, Jimmy Ellis, and Michael Dokes, each the possessor of large punching power. Every day he exposed his flanks (his kidneys) to devastating punches.

Conclusion: Ali should have quit.

I'm proud of standing up for my convictions. I'm unhappy to see that I was right. A brilliant comet like a starlit ride came crashing down to earth. It happens in the movies, politics, the military, and yes, heavyweight championship fighting.

Painful as it was, if I had to do all over again, I would have jumped after Manila and had a chance to save him.

✗✗✗✗✗✗

Now suffering from Parkinson's disease, Ali plods on, shaking, shuffling, and mumbling, an object of pity.

How does Ali respond to this? Just like he did against Sonny Liston, Joe Frazier, and George Foreman. He meets his illness head on and will not buckle under; he fights it bell to bell, travels the world speaking until he can't say another word, and then his wife or Howard Bingham, his photographer and confidant, speaks for him.

His irresistible spirit still shines. A few years ago at a heavyweight championship fight, we saw each other and embraced—me, choked up with a tear; Ali, with a sly smile. He hugged me tightly, and mumbled in my ear, "You still a ghetto nigger," and we both laughed, remembering a day in his penthouse suite at the Fontainebleau Hotel in Miami Beach when we planned his visit to my little ghetto clinic. The gang and at least 12 ne'er-do-well hangers-on were discussing how many limos they would need because they were, they said, "ghetto niggers."

I got hot. I didn't need an appearance. I wanted Ali to come himself in a taxi and simply sit in my office and say nice things to each patient as they came to my desk. No money would change hands, no T-shirts, and no glossy photos; just Muhammad Ali being his lovable self.

The argument grew hot until I finally blew up. "There isn't *one* ghetto nigger in this room, including you, Ali. It's been 15 years since you used to hang in my office, bragging about what you were going to do to Liston."

Ali stood up.

"That's right! Doc's right!" he said, followed by more grumbling from his gang about their rights as ghetto niggers.

"The only one in this room that's a ghetto nigger is me," I said, and I think I was the only Caucasian present!

"Ten hours a day, six days a week. You people probably have never even seen the Miami ghetto unless you were driving through it in a limo!" I shouted.

Ali jumped as if he'd been shot. He was clapping, shrieking, laughing.

"He's right! Doc's the ghetto nigger here," he declared.

Ali came to the clinic, all right, but he attracted an ABC-TV truck. Goodbye to *that* idea! He meant well, but Ali was famous, you know.

✗✗✗✗✗✗

I have been with Ali through his great moments in the ring, but the highlight for me was the Atlanta Olympics when, incredibly enough, he was chosen to light the torch. As I sat in the audience, I prayed as hard as I could that Ali would be able to climb the steps, hold the torch steady, and ignite the flame. I wasn't alone. I could feel the entire crowd praying with me, "Oh God, please don't let him drop the torch. Please, don't let him embarrass himself."

This was classic Ali. Give him an impossible task, and he will complete it.

How does he do it? I don't know. "Ali's luck" I call it, but that seems too easy, too trite.

The answer is that I believe Muhammad Ali is God's chosen child. God looks after him and protects him, because he is made in His image and radiates His glow.

That's my explanation. Do you have a better one?

CHAPTER 6

Luisita Sevilla: My Fourth Love

The ultimate partnership in life is one we make with a stranger, to share a life, to make a family, and to find comfort and serenity in the company of another person. Where is such person to be found? How can you predict who is the right person?

My case was old, but not unique. It's called love at first sight, and as these things go, it happened to me at a most unforeseen moment. Let me set the scene.

By 1969, I was in the fourth year of waiting for the decision of the Supreme Court, where my querimonious second wife had taken our case. Her high-paid attorneys argued that adultery in front of the children was not a reason to award the kids to the father. They lost their argument. My pal Petula Clark called from Yugoslavia, where she was making a movie, to say the headline made history in the Dubrovnik's newspaper, and started with the quote, "Notwithstanding the sexual habits of sea otters, moose and elks, the human race is quite different." They lost. I won.

During these hard four years I had been going with a beautiful ex-Miss Florida contestant, who was in her mid-30s and had one son from a marriage to a wealthy French media mogul who had newspapers, magazines, radio, and TV stations all over Haiti.

The woman was very sweet and well mannered. Her demeanor was half old South and half European. She was talented in that she was qualified to teach piano. She owned a very large house, and her son was a well-behaved, bright kid.

Twice before, I slid slowly into marriage. I never rushed precipitously to the altar screaming, "I've got to have you." Unfortunately, four years had gone by, and the bright burning light of "I've got to have you" had dimmed. I was sliding into a third marriage. I was happy with my choice. I thought she was perfect for me; my kids—Evelyn, Dawn, and Ferdie—liked her; even my cat liked her.

So what happened?

It was a dark, murky afternoon, and the Dolphins were playing the Patriots in New England. It was a very close game. I sat in my apartment watching the game with Gil Clancy, a boxing pal, and Hector Mendez, an Argentine madman and boxing promoter.

Hector had a contract for Jimmy Ellis to fight Goyo Peralta, a good Argentine heavyweight, for the championship. He had planned to promote the fight in Uruguay, because he could not, under any condition, promote the fight in Argentina where boxing was run with an iron fist by people like Tito Lectore. Hector got the principals to sign, paid our advance, and then proceeded to stupidly change the venue to Buenos Aires. Goodbye fight, which was a horrible mistake for Hector, because Peralta had a veritable lock-cinch to beat Ellis.

Hector also held a contract for the popular international band Los Chavales de España to appear in a carnival in Brazil, and at that moment they were playing in Miami at Prilas, the best Cuban nightclub restaurant in town. He wanted me to accompany him and Gil to the club.

"Nah, I've seen Los Chavales a 100 times or more. They're good, but not that good."

"They have two dancers who look like twins they're so beautiful," said Hector hopefully.

Gil asked me to go because it figured to be a night of Spanish and no English being spoken. I liked Gil and felt sorry for him, so I decided what the hell, I'd go.

The lights dimmed, and a lovely Spanish song, "Madrid," began, played by French horn. As the lights came up, there stood two incredibly lovely Spanish girls in beautiful tight-fitting Madroleño costumes, an elegant long dress from the turn of the century. They were both stunning, and so alike that I assumed they were twins. The show was great; the girls had performed several flamenco and Spanish classical dances. They would stop the show.

After the show, Hector sat huddled with the manager of the band, and Gil and I went to the bar where we sat at a back table to view the action. Nothing much was happening. A few bottom-heavy Cuban hookers were talking prices with some potbellied Johns, and I was getting fidgety when, walking in front of us, came this incredible vision of loveliness. She wore a sparkling top and peach-colored pants. She was still in her stage makeup, so she looked unreal in her beauty.

Now I must stop here to show how serendipity, my old friend, worked.

One of my best friends, Barry Sinco, was a gambling casino manager, whom I met years ago as a reluctant pharmaceutical representative. He was tall, handsome, and his highest aspiration in life was to be a standup comic. He had only one drawback. He was not funny onstage. So he toured the world of big-time gambling, and wherever our paths intersected—Monte Carlo, Vegas, Puerto Rico, or Atlantic City—we would party. Barry Sinco and I went through a regiment of gorgeous girls. One day he came through Miami, and said to me, "Ferdie, I've met the girl you're going to marry. Once you meet her, it's all over, pal."

Barry Sinco knew I had been going with a nice girl for four years and had every intention of marrying her as soon as my divorce formally ended. He waved off my objections.

"You'll see. This girl has every one of the qualities you like in your women, plus she is better looking than anyone we've been around. And she can cook Spanish, American, or Mexican food. She's an American from Denver of Spanish descent; she spent time in Seville learning to dance like she does. She is from a great family. Never been married, no strings on her, no children, she's a very creative person, the best flamenco dancer I've ever seen."

"Whoa," I said, impressed with the blast of superlatives, "if she's so great, you marry her."

"I don't qualify. If anybody wins her, it's because they speak and act Spanish."

Time went by, and naturally I forgot about the Spanish beauty who had overwhelmed Barry Sinco.

Now, as she strode purposely to the exit, Barry's story flashed into my brain.

"If you don't go talk to her, I will," said Gil, who appreciated beauty as much as I did.

I caught up with her as she reached the door and hailed her. She gave me a kind but frosty stare. I blurted out, "You are a friend of Barry Sinco. He told me if you were ever in Miami, I'm to show you around and get whatever you need."

Her beautiful face softened, and she smiled her radiant smile. God, she was inhumanely beautiful. She spoke to me in English, not Spanish, and we began a long conversation, which has lasted until today. We went out to get a bite, and spent most of the night having a delightfully fun and laughter-filled evening.

I went home and couldn't sleep. Barry was right. I had to have this girl as a wife.

But I had a great girlfriend. The poor girl had done nothing wrong; she was sweet, patient, and supportive as I slogged my way through a messy divorce. I couldn't afford a third mistake.

My first marriage to Paula had been a good match, but it had come at a time of maximum stress trying to make ends meet. It wore us both out, and we both agreed to a friendly divorce. The second marriage was a rebound marriage. I found a gorgeous showgirl who looked like my first wife. She had saved a bit of money, enough to pay for my senior year and internship, and I caved in and slid into another marriage. This one proved to be very difficult. The good thing that came from it was that we had had two children, Dawn and Ferdie Jim, in addition to her daughter, Evelyn. I had won everything in the settlement, but I swore never to get married again unless I absolutely felt like I had to.

For six weeks, I juggled both my girlfriend and Luisita, neither one knew about the other. Finally, Luisita had to go with the troupe to Puerto Rico for a month. During that time, I decided to solve the impasse.

There was no easy way. I had to do some cold surgery. I would badly hurt someone I had truly loved and who had done nothing to deserve this painful fate. Being a master at disengaging at this time of my life, I had learned that the act must be sudden, terminal, and brutally final, so that the offended party must hate you, despise you, and not want you back. Once out, there can be no second thoughts, no going back. From Argentina came the invitation from Hector Mendez to save me and provide a foolproof exit from the nasty situation. Also, at this exact time a cholera epidemic hit the children of the ghetto. We ran out of serum. I was fighting Washington to get the serum I needed to save them.

As I was to leave for Argentina and the Ellis fight, my intended called, worried that I was getting cold feet as her mother and grandmother suspected, and she wanted reassurance.

I exploded.

"I'm in the midst of a cholera epidemic. I'm on the phone to Washington to get more serum, and you call me with that? I'm hanging up. If you call back, you'll never see me again."

I hung up.

The trip to Argentina took two weeks, and in the interim she'd get the message. My friends told her about my infatuation with Luisita, and painful as it was, the affair was over. I was devastated because I had never done anything intentionally bad to hurt anyone in my life.

My difficult decision proved extremely correct. I married lovely Luisita, had a gorgeous daughter, Tina, and am still living happily ever after.

The girl, after a terrible phase, recovered, met a decent Spanish businessman, married, had a daughter, and has lived a quiet happy life. For that I am supremely happy, because she didn't deserve that hurt.

Marriage with Luisita Sevilla, a.k.a. Karen Maestas, has been a seamless dream. A happy marriage is one is which two people melt into one, each more interested in their own partner's happiness and welfare than in their own. Eventually as time flies by you find you have become one person with two heads. You respect and help the partner maintain her identity, help her grow and succeed.

In our case we are both creative people—growing, ever pushing ourselves to bigger and better successes.

I often say that had it not been for Luisita's faith and prodding, I would not have become the artist I am today. She encouraged me to paint large paintings, some that have sold for as much as $40,000.

She encouraged me to write. She helps me type and edit all of my books. She is the business head and pilot light of Pacheco Creative. And yet, she still dances. Even at the age of nearly 60, she has the style, grace, and fire necessary to dance flamenco, called *duende*.

Today, our little empire totters along propelled by her incredible energy and intelligence; she has structured a beautiful website, ferdiepacheco.com. She books my art exhibits and speeches and helps me to do research on all of my books.

And she is still the most beautiful girl I know. I recognize the fact that I am shallow in that way, but God help me, I do so appreciate a beautiful face.

So love at first sight. Does it exist? Does it work? It did for me.

CHAPTER 7

Tits for Television

It was dark in the little dressing room. The only light was a lamp, covered by a wet towel, and the only sound was the deep gasp for air followed by guttural groans from an exhausted fighter. Slowly, with a giant hand still taped for combat, he painfully pulled up a bottle of Gatorade to his swollen lips and let the orange liquid flow over them into his dry mouth.

Lou Esa, the "White Hope" of Miami's Fifth Street Gym, lay on an undersized rubbing table, his huge feet hanging over the end, trying to get up enough energy to make it to the showers and feel the cold water restore his black-and-blue bruised body.

Just as he was starting to breathe normally again, abandoning the thought of suicide, the dressing room door sprang open and in walked the ebullient godfather of Miami boxing, Chris Dundee. The best description of Chris that comes to mind is he looked like a humped-over Groucho Marx wearing boxing gloves.

"Wow! What a great fight!" Chris said, thumping Esa on the shoulder.

Esa groaned.

"Tell you what, I got a great surprise for you 'cuz you done good," Chris beamed.

"Like what? Are you gonna give me $200 more?" Esa said, always looking to get paid what he was worth.

"Nah," Chris skipped lightly over the possibility that he might have to part with a buck. "Next month I'm putting you on top. You're gonna be the top draw."

Chris stepped back anxiously to let all of the goodness of that reward sink into Esa's exhausted mind.

"For $200 more," Lou said, not a man to let a good idea go easily. "At least $200."

"And more," Chris said, rubbing his hands together and expecting appreciation from Esa.

"Wait a minute," Esa said, his mind clearing on hearing Chris give in so easily on a $200 raise. Red flags flew in his mind as he wondered what the catch was. Painfully, he pulled himself to a sitting position.

"Just wait a minute …. Top of the show? Does that mean I have to fight 10 rounds?"

The thought paralyzed him. God, he had just barely made four.

"Ten rounds, or *less,*" Chris purred. "It's up to you, champ. Knock the sucker out in two, and you'll get the same dough."

"Yeah, but suppose it goes 10? Christ, I can't even go four without dyin'. How the hell do you think I can go 10?"

"Look, kid, you get tired with a four-round fight, because you just get three minutes of rest between rounds. With a 10-round fight, you get nine minutes of rest." Chris moved in closer in a nose-to-nose confrontation and whispered with the intensity and wisdom of a Mafia don. "Nine minutes of rest." He knowingly clapped the big man on the shoulder as if he had just revealed the secret of the universe.

I looked at Esa's manager, Murray Gaby, and his trainer, Dwayne Simpson, and it was all we could do to keep from busting out laughing. Esa just blinked.

"Bullshit! You go 10 and rest for nine, not me. No way! Fuck you and your nine minutes."

In the end, not even Chris could convince Esa to try any more than four. That was no way to get to the golden halls of the heavyweight championship fights, so Esa dawdled along at the four-round level, with no hope of moving into the big bucks. It was a wasted opportunity at heavy money.

Years flew by and Esa's precarious reputation spread throughout the boxing world. Ask any of the gray men of the Fifth Street Gym College of Cardinals and they would give you this appraisal of him: big, white, good-looking kid. Can punch for two rounds, and then he's through. He was never in shape, couldn't take a hard rap. He was a real bow-wow.

✗✗✗✗✗✗

Big Lou was a marketable commodity known as *the* (never 'an') *opponent.*

For a big guy, he had a disarming, self-deprecating wit and the ability to laugh his way through anything. At some point, he tired of being a ladies' man and picked the best-looking girl in his harem, a Cuban-American named Julie. She was unbelievably beautiful, with a fine, full Cuban figure on a five-foot-eight frame. Julie could easily win any beauty contest, and she had won her share, when she abandoned whatever ambitions beauty queens have and opted for a home and children with Esa.

Julie and Lou were a golden couple. Wherever they went, they stood out, even more so because he took his mother-in-law with them, who, unbelievably enough, was even better looking than Julie. So Esa walked in a room towering above everyone and was bookended by two gorgeous women.

In time Julie became very critical of her appearance and decided she was deficient in breast tissue. She had no tits, at least not sufficient enough for her. Esa couldn't care less. His area of erogenous interest was on the dorsal side of her body, so he never took a good look at the ventral side of his curvaceous wife. They never interested him, so, in his mind, they didn't matter.

Julie's lack of tits got to be a serious bone of contention until she put her foot down. In order to make life livable, she needed boobs. So Esa came to me, because I took care of all of the boxers' medical problems. My best friend was a world-renowned plastic surgeon by the name of Howard Gordon, who fixed boxing injuries, fractured hands, and broken noses for free. Breasts, however, were another matter. He'd have to charge, and even with Esa's professional discount it came to $5,000, an impossible sum of money for a four-round fighter.

Esa was well connected. Murray Gaby, his manager in Miami Beach, was a very interesting man who had boxing deep in his soul. He didn't need to, God knows, but Gaby loved to manage fighters. Initially he fought on the boxing team at Idaho State and then came to Miami to turn pro at the Fifth Street Gym. Gaby's real name was Gaby, but the gray men said that sounded poofy, so they changed it to Marty Kaplan to reflect his Jewish roots. He did well and went undefeated, but his hands crumbled, and because he was known as a puncher, he quit. He had also trained as a painter under the famous German artist, George

Grosz. So after his boxing career, he was able to find a lucrative position in the advertising business.

Esa had a great corner: a fashionable, well-dressed artist with a beaten-up face as a manager. For a trainer he had a hilarious cracker kid named Dwayne Simpson, who had fought for Gaby and who had the sense of humor to write "Goodnight, Irene" on the soles of his boxing slippers. That alone tells you he didn't go far as a boxer, but he was a good trainer. Esa also had me (all modesty aside), Muhammad Ali's doctor.

Chris Dundee put out feelers, and soon big-time New York promoter, Bob Arum, called. He needed a body to get knocked out, and the safe choice was the tall, handsome Esa.

"Lou's your man!" shouted Chris and Gaby.

"How much?" Arum asked guardedly.

"Five thousand dollars," Gaby replied, his heart beating fast and thinking about tits, plastic surgeons, and withholding taxes, "in cash."

After the usual crying and mewling died down, Arum agreed to $5,000 and plane tickets. The fight was to take place on November 18, 1977, in Las Vegas at one of the big hotels, and it would be televised by CBS. It would also showcase two brothers, Leon and Michael Spinks.

"Who are we fighting?" I asked, as if it made a difference.

"Some farmer from Carolina, or Memphis, or someplace," Gaby answered. "A raw talent. We could get lucky."

Murray never learned how to look reality in the face.

I figured we had no chance going in, because if a curmudgeon like Arum was willing to put $5,000 down on a four-round opponent, then he was absolutely sure the fight was a mismatch, and Esa had no chance. Chris would guarantee it! Sixteen straight knockouts.

When we arrived in Las Vegas with our wives, we took Esa to a roadside motel a short distance from where we were staying. We figured that, after roadwork and a meal, he would welcome a good night's sleep where nobody would bother him. Then we went to our hotel, which was one of the top glitzy money-making palaces to grace The Strip. On our way to our rooms we made reservations for dinner at the luxurious main dining room. We were so caught up in the electric whirlwind spinning around us that Gaby and I forgot our most salient rule: Never leave Lou Esa alone, in a motel room, in a strange town. He just couldn't be trusted. His wise-cracking, devilish way gave him a natural affinity for pissing off the men in blue.

We had finished our meal and were awaiting our espresso when we heard an uproar from the far side of the room. Security is tight in Vegas casinos, so we paid the disruption scant attention. But a moment later, a mob of policemen came pushing by our table. Among the hurly-burly of big-muscled cops was the towering figure of Esa, in handcuffs, no less, being dragged toward a waiting paddy wagon.

"I'm innocent!" Esa bellowed as he passed our table. "It's police brutality!"

That remark fetched him a smart clout on the head with a rubber truncheon.

Gaby scrambled from the table, yelling, "He's innocent!"

I immediately phoned Bob. He met us at the hotel, and we raced to the jail, hoping we could get there before Esa complicated whatever trouble he'd gotten himself into.

It took us until 4 a.m. to spring him. I hasten to point out that staying in jail and getting whacked around all night is not the ideal way to train for a fight, but Esa didn't seem fazed.

"What's the trouble?" he asked innocently. "I got all day to sleep."

Greatly relieved, but sorry that we had missed our reservations to see Keely Smith in the lounge, we went back to our hotel and I fell into a restless sleep while Gaby was, no doubt, twitching in excitement at the prospect that Esa would provide us with an upset.

At the weigh-in that evening, I ran across an old friend from the Ali days, CBS star commentator Brent Musburger, for whom I have great respect. He was much younger than I was, with a college boy look and a nice, warm personality. He handed me a challenge by inviting me to the delicatessen to try to fit a six-inch-tall pastrami sandwich in my mouth. I went, not for the challenge, but because I had an ulterior motive.

Besides recounting Ali stories with Musburger, I wanted to tell him about my first book, *The Fight Doctor*, that had recently been published. In my naivete, I was hoping he could plug it on CBS. Ever the gentleman, Musburger assured me he could. He'd work it into the best round of the Esa fight. Then he gave me his best "Would I lie to you?" manner.

I innocently told him what I thought would be best.

"Between rounds one and two, there's likely to be a knockout. Esa'll say bye-bye."

To his credit, Musburger broke out a pad and felt-tipped pen and wrote all this down. I had taken pains to carry a copy of the book with me, which I left with the courtly Musburger, and walked out feeling proud of having nailed a nationwide endorsement on CBS by no less a star than Brent Musburger! Of course, knowing what I know now of television commentating, I am embarrassed to relate how hard I bit on that con, because CBS wouldn't be caught dead televising a four-round fight on an undercard, especially not Lou Esa against a dirt farmer. Musburger had no intention of plugging the book. He just wanted to watch me make a fool of myself, flat-out jiving me by patting me on the head and sending me on my way. I felt like an unregistered dog.

Talk about naïve. I knew all there was to know about the dark underbelly of boxing, but I was a dumb rube when it came to television.

We were in the ring at Caesar's Palace when the crowd started filing in. When the place was about half filled, I saw this huge, heavily muscled black guy coming up the ring stairs.

"Is that our opponent?" I asked urgently, grabbing Gaby by the arm.

He looked over his shoulder and gave out a matter-of-fact, "Yeah."

"Christ Almighty!" I started jumping around like Kermit the Frog. "Don't you know who that is? That's John Tate, the next Heavyweight Champion of the World! He's a monster!"

There was a flicker of awareness in Esa's eyes, so I decided to level with him.

"Lou, I want you to fight with everything you got in round one. You might get lucky and knock out this guy."

Esa could really punch when he was fresh, before exhaustion immobilized his arm, and he went down like a sinking battleship.

I came up nose to nose with his huge face.

"If he's still here for round two, look for a soft spot to land, then dive for cover and don't get up." I emphasized what I was saying with a point of my finger.

He seemed not to hear me, but replied, "No problemo, Doc. I'm knockin' out this motherfucker."

The crowd got its money's worth in the first round. Esa won; at least it looked that way. Then he staggered back to the stool and plopped his heavy body down, gasping for breath. His eyes rolled around in his head.

"What round is it?" he asked.

"What round?" I said, disbelievingly. "What round? For Chrissake, that was the first round!"

"Shit."

The second round was unreasonably fast. Tate came out and pole-axed Esa, who was riveted to the canvas, unable to raise his arms to fend off the big lumbering punches. He fell like a collapsing beach chair, one part at a time. It was ugly.

Gaby and I jumped into the ring. Esa, on his knees, was taller than I was standing up.

"Where are we?" I asked him to see how far out he was.

"Somewhere up there in the rafters," he answered, and I couldn't help but agree with him.

So that is how Esa managed 17 straight knockouts.

Later that night, while I was in the dressing room getting my gear together, a pimple-faced runner from CBS burst in.

"Brent wants you at ringside," he said. "Hurry up, we're about to go on."

"Oh boy," I thought. "Brent is going to keep his promise and plug my book!"

I rushed down to ringside in my white doctor's smock, and an aide handed me a headset and a microphone and sat me beside Musburger, who was into his pitch about my book *The Fight Doctor.* Then we went to a commercial.

"I need an expert analyst," Musburger said breathlessly. "I hear you know how to do this."

I nodded the affirmative. I had helped Howard Cosell many nights during our Ali fights. Mostly I wrote notes of my observations and insights, pushing them to Cosell. Angelo Dundee and Gil Clancy did the same thing, which helped build Cosell's reputation as a top-notch commentator. His fans thought he really knew boxing, but what he really knew was broadcasting and little or nothing about boxing.

It says a lot for Musburger's intelligence and character that at least he knew he was out of his league commentating on boxing. He couldn't do a credible job by himself, and he knew it. And because Gil Clancy, who was doing a great job for CBS, was tied up at home taking care of his sick wife, there was no one there but me.

Ta-da! I was in the right place at the right time, and my star was born. Well, maybe not a star, but at least I was credible, could talk a good line, and knew all about boxing.

The first fight was Michael Spinks against Gary Summerhays. There was a great difference between the two Spinks brothers. Michael could fight! He was sensational, as his long and successful career would show. Leon was a one-trick pony. He had strength, energy, and the rabid attack psychology of a U.S. Marine, which he had been, but little else.

Back in New York, Barry Frank, the executive producer of CBS, listened closely.

The next fight, Leon Spinks versus Alfio Righetti, was coming up, and Frank made a snap decision.

"Whoever the fuck that is sitting next to Brent in the box, keep him there."

And that was my start in television. Call it serendipity, fate, or pure luck, but opportunity met necessity, and I was hired to commentate fights for CBS.

The fight was a huge yawn. I figured it was because Leon was scheduled to fight Ali if he got past this tub of spaghetti. Leon had fought only six fights! It was a shame to put him in with Ali, yet I felt, even then, that Leon could beat Ali, and I said so. That was a daring statement for live TV. The reason I said it was that I knew what pathetic shape Ali was in. He wasn't training at all, and on every level, he was falling apart. His brain was damaged and getting worse; his kidneys were so shot that he was passing whole blood and lines of kidney tubule cells as well.

Frank, still watching from his New York office, had it all planned out, telling his assistant, "The Doc will work the Ali–Spinks fight with Brent."

He was so sure of the quality of the event that he ventured a prediction.

"It'll be an Emmy," he said.

And he was right. We won an Emmy for that show. In my first primetime fight, and my second time with Musburger, we won an Emmy! *That* was easy.

And did Musburger plug my book? Yes he did, bless him, in both fights. I learned to really love that guy—he was a class act.

Now you can see how my career got flung into play by the pinball flaps and hit many different targets along the way, but even though they seemed disconnected, they all came together at one point where I came out a winner. Stick with me, and I'll tell you how serendipity worked to hand me an Emmy for my second telecast.

But first, I can't just leave Lou Esa lying in a bed of pain. Actually Esa got out of trouble and did bring home the $5,000. Julie got her operation, but nature took a strange turn.

Esa had a Cuban friend named Julio, who was small in stature and worshipped Esa. Julio worked as Esa's go-fer and slave. Esa was not a normal stay-at-home husband. He delegated all husbandly duties to Julio, who was happy to walk in the footsteps of the goddess Julie. Esa was a sociopath, which resulted in tiffs with the law and intermittent incarceration. It was during one of his many incarcerations that Esa got a letter informing him that the lovely Julie had divorced him and that she was marrying Julio! Esa and Julie had a set of twin daughters, and luckily, Esa understood it was better to have a calm, quiet home than a jailbird father, so he took the news quite well. He now lives in Spain with his two grown daughters—at least technically he lives in Spain.

I received a nice, long letter from Esa recently. I hadn't heard from him since Tate knocked him into the rafters, but in typical Esa fashion in writing about his crime he said, "If the judge was sentencing me on dumbness, I would have gotten life."

Talk about serendipity.

✗✗✗✗✗✗

There had been a rustle of concerned voices over Ali's obvious physical deterioration, with my loud mouth leading the way. I had begged him to retire and told him if he didn't he could risk serious brain damage, possibly even death. And my on-air prediction that an out-of-shape Ali would lose his title was making nice publicity for CBS. Everybody was happy to have me.

Frank orchestrated the show, using Angelo Dundee as analyst for the first fight, Gil Clancy for the second, an ex-champion welterweight from Mexico for the third, and Musburger and me for the last one.

I arrived, checked in, and was told to report to a production meeting. I was absolutely ignorant of how a TV production was orchestrated, so I went in with an open mind.

"After all," I figured, "what did I have to do with their production outside of being there for the opening bell, and then I was on my own."

Nobody had told me what to say, or how to say it. Hell, I really didn't know how I was going to take it, seeing Ali in the ring, probably taking a beating, without me standing by, ready to tend his wounds. I loved that big guy. It was going to be hard.

The production meeting convened on a raised stage where the show's opening would take place. This was my first face-to-face meeting with Frank. He was short, dynamic, and very pleasant. Even when standing still, he seemed to vibrate with creative energy. The president of CBS, Bob Wussler, was there, too. He was a tall New York Athletic Club type of snob—gracious but a bit condescending. The way Wussler was twirling his unopened pen, I could tell he wasn't comfortable without a drink in his hand. He didn't say much, just left the hands-on management to Frank, who seemed to have every facet of the program under his control.

"The first thing will be Brent introducing the show and the commentators," Frank said. "Then the overview will be turned over to our super-anchor Jack Whitaker."

So far so good, I thought. That would give me time to think of something to say, write it down, and see how much time I have to say it.

Musburger sat us all down and gave a safe, generic hello to Vegas, touched on what the audience was about to see, and then turned to Jack Whitaker, the ultimate voice of truth. No bullshit, no sales pitch, Whitaker leveled with the audience. At the time CBS was trying to figure some way to compete with Howard Cosell's ABC hit show *Tell It Like It Is.*

Whitaker, looking unnecessarily smug, began talking with a real smirk to his voice, "You can forget the first three fights. They're basically mismatches."

Huh? I leaned forward to give him the fisheye. How does he know that for sure? You never really know how it's going to turn out until the bell rings. Plus you are kicking your network in the balls. I looked at Frank and Wussler, who were smiling angelically. What was going on here? Were they just trying to mimic Cosell? If they were, it was a damned poor job.

Whitaker shifted in his chair and gave the camera his "tell the truth" look. "As far as Ali's fight, the only real fight here tonight will be in the ratings between Ali and *Charlie's Angels.*"

ABC's *Charlie's Angels* happened to be our opposition in that time slot. It was a very hot show at the time, and featured Farrah Fawcett, who alone could knock us out of the box. Ali in a walkover fight with an inexperienced kid was no match for the shapely *Charlie's Angels,* and Whitaker had just told the viewers that without batting an eyelash. CBS had invested $2 million to hear their ace commentator tell the audience they were a bunch of lunkheads for even watching the fight at all.

I actually thought he was kidding. It had to be a send-up, a gag of some kind, but no one was laughing. And Wussler was beaming like a headlight. Then something snapped in me, and I got really angry. The thought that he could take something as powerful as a championship boxing match and compare it to the same puff-and-panties mentality of *Charlie's Angels* was beyond me. There were no buxom broads in stilettos out there in the ring, and I was as mad as a bull in the box. He finally clapped shut, but not before dissing Ali.

Musburger gave me a thin smile.

"Well, Doc, how do you see the Ali–Spinks fight?"

I leaned over slightly and put my hand on Whitaker's arm, trying to look professional about it all.

"Did you really mean what you just said, or are you just kidding around?" He didn't respond, so I shrugged my shoulders a bit and began, "Tonight we're going to see one of the greatest upsets of the past two decades. Leon Spinks, the ex-Marine, with seven fights, will out-work, outfight, and outlast the great Muhammad Ali.

"Ali is woefully out of shape. He has trained six days for this fight and is physically falling apart. Besides the brain damage he's been sustaining, he now has major kidney damage. He hasn't taken this fight seriously. He thinks he can phone this one in.

"So, if you want to see boxing history in the making, stay tuned. It's going to be an evening you won't want to miss."

Whitaker didn't even blink. He stood up, put his headset on the desk, and left without a word as I sat there watching him. I walked over to Frank and Wussler, who were congratulating themselves on a spot well done. I didn't care who these people were, or what their titles were, I wanted to be heard.

I looked at Wussler in his European tuxedo and started in without fanfare.

"Are you going to let Whitaker get away with that? Not only is he wrong, but he's insulting you and CBS. It's costing $2 million, and your guy is telling the audience they're all fools for watching it."

Boy, was I green. He put his arm around my shoulder as if pacifying an unruly child.

"Doc, we are in an age of truth in television. We want … we even encourage our people to speak the truth, even if it hurts."

Well, I had never heard anything that ridiculous and had no way of countering his thinking, so I said, "Okay. If that's the game, I'll play it out, but remember—Ali will lose tonight and there's gonna be a whole lot of people watching *Charlie's Angels* when he does."

I went back to the box without another word. This wasn't the kind of boxing world I was from.

We were now ringside. I was standing next to Musburger, and I must say, we looked great with our black tuxes reflecting the harsh arena lights. The countdown began …three …two …one … *showtime!* The producer screeched in my ear. Musburger leaned in to me as we waited for the red light to go on.

"Now, Doc, this is 20 million viewers," he said in his most serious tone. "Don't choke on me."

Boy, that was just what I needed to hear. What motivation, what comfort. When one of my patients stopped breathing and I couldn't get him started, then I might choke, or when more blood was coming out than going in, I could get worried, but this … this was dog shit. Here I am saying to America that Ali is about to lose his title!

The fight went exactly as I'd predicted. I had moments when I got a little emotional, because we were witnessing a disgrace. Ali should not have been fighting anymore. I cringed as I watched an amateur kid pummel the greatest fighter of all time. Ali's untenable past had finally caught up with him.

Finally, it was all over. Ali had lost, and everybody was crying. Even Angelo's wife, Helen, was mad.

"Why don't you go tell that kid to quit?" she asked her husband. "Do like Doc and refuse to be with him if he fights again."

Poor Angelo, intimidated by his wife, went up and mumbled those words to Ali, but without much conviction. Ali just looked at him through tired eyes and managed a "Yeah, yeah," but they both knew there would be other nights, and Angelo would always be with Ali. They started together; they would finish together.

The upshot of my performance was that CBS hired me in 1979, and for about a year, I commentated fights with Angelo as my broadcast partner. That was a terrible idea, because Angelo had taught me all I knew about boxing, so we were always saying the same things. We couldn't disagree because we were seeing the same thing through the same eyes.

✗✗✗✗✗✗

As soon as I got home from the Ali telecast, I was called to see a patient at the Cricket Club, a chi-chi club for adult delinquents. I was the doctor for clubs like that, the Palm Bay, and Zef Bufman's theatrical companies. Through those connections, I had made a good friend in Vic Jarmel. He had been an agent for International Creative Management, ICM, assigned to take Artie Shaw and his band on tour and later assigned to look after Jackie Gleason and his many needs while in Miami Beach.

Jarmel took me to lunch to meet his ex-boss and his wife. There was no purpose to the lunch, no objective. It was just a relaxed lunch in a great club. His ex-boss at ICM was Buddy Howe, who was a small ex-vaudevillian, ex-hoofer, and acrobat. Unlike most heads of agencies, he had kind eyes and an ability to relax and enjoy a good story. He wanted to hear about Ali. Who didn't?

For once in my life, I was more impressed with his wife. She was now in her 60s, and she was gorgeous. I learned that she had been

Howe's partner in vaudeville and that she carried the act with her off-the-wall comedy until reality set in when Howe turned into her manager and then agent, and she became Jean Carroll.

I found the two to be wonderful company, great listeners, and when Carroll felt like it, a great, funny storyteller.

Over that winter, we became close. They ate at our house and loved Luisita and my daughter Tina, who was very young then and terminally cute.

When it was time for them to go back to The Big Apple, Carroll, who also had great eye for talent, told Howe to take me on. I needed representation.

I had been doing a fight-by-fight deal with CBS. I should have had an agent to negotiate that. I had a serious novel, *The Lector*, for which I needed a high-powered agent. I was doing fine art and needed a New York art show. And Carroll fell in love with "Sweet Sam," my Christmas card short story, in which Norman Lear also had shown such interest. She saw it as a Hallmark season special, which is exactly what it was. In short, Buddy Howe, the emperor, should adopt me.

As their behest, I went to New York City. It was freezing that year. I stayed with Howe and Carroll at their apartment while he put the humongous ICM machinery at my disposal.

I learned then that, contrary to what one would think, it is not to your advantage to be brought in by the top boss as this year's project. For one thing, Howe was a tough boss. He expected results. So I was seen as a ticking land mine. No one wanted the job. They knew they would fail, and they would get kicked in the teeth by Howe.

One morning, Howe called all excited, and told me to come right away and bring my huge novel, *The Lector*. He had ICM's top agent waiting to see us.

Howe walked me to her office. The sight of Howe and me walking through the offices prompted an exodus, something like the parting of the Red Sea.

"She did the *Jaws* deal. Millions! Millions!" Buddy kept saying excitedly.

We stepped into her office, and I thought I stepped into a time warp. We were in the 18th century; the colonials were rebelling against the crown.

All over her office were artifacts of the Revolutionary War, and she was knitting an American flag with 13 stars. She looked as old as George Washington. Okay maybe Thomas Jefferson. Boy, was I in the wrong place!

Howe did a glowing introduction, which basically translated to "Here is a book I want to get published. See to it!" Howe signaled for me to plop the two huge volumes of more than 750 pages on her desk.

"Oh, God," she groaned, "I'm suppose to schlep all that [shit] on the train?"

Right at that moment, I knew I was toast. Howe or no Howe, she rejected it right there.

"Well, if it will be of any help, I'll reduce it to microfilm, and you can take it home in a handbag."

"Is that sarcasm or irony?" she gritted out.

"Somewhere between both." I then tipped my hat and left.

And so it went. Howe tried public speaking dates, appearances on talk shows, *People* magazine articles, a solid contract with CBS (they died laughing), and a really hard try at getting "Sweet Sam" made as a movie.

Zilch. Zero. Abject and total failure.

Still, it was a start in the creative world of New York in the 1970s. I learned an awful lot about showbiz from Howe and Carroll. She was a great booster and an honest critic. When things were very funny, she whooped and hollered. If they didn't click, she told you so. Carroll was what every writer needs: an honest critic.

Unfortunately, Howe died of leukemia in 1981. I was devastated. I still miss his wonderful company. Thankfully, we still have the beautiful, witty Jean Carroll, who comes to see us every winter. She's still funny as hell.

✗✗✗✗✗✗

As it happened to me all my life, in 1980 one door closed (ICM) and another opened (IMG). Serendipity. Unthinking and unknowing, I stood still and acquired the help of one of sport's most powerful and knowledgeable men, Barry Frank.

Frank, the man who discovered me at CBS, was fired—or quit, depending on whom you asked. Some say he called tennis matches winner take all when, in fact, both players got paid. He walked away, and CBS was the loser, because Frank was a TV genius.

In my own soft-hearted and naïve way, I felt bad for Frank. I pictured him out there in the vast wasteland of dejected television executives with nowhere to go and bills to pay. I knew his true genius was unappreciated, so I wrote him a long letter of encouragement and offered him my support in any way I could. After all, I was very well connected after my long tour with Ali, so I offered to contact my sources and get him a deserving position, an ambassadorship in Guatemala, perhaps.

He must have laughed himself to death over a highball when he got that letter. Hell, I thought Frank had been relegated to Siberia, when in actuality he entertained all kinds of offers. Everybody wanted to hire the Sammy Glick of American sports TV. Frank landed on his feet as a partner in the biggest sports promotion agency in America, IMG. In no time he was bigger than ever, and here I had felt bad for him! Good intentions are sometimes, though infrequently, rewarded. When Frank joined IMG, he called and wanted to represent me.

That was the break I needed. NBC was going to the Moscow Summer Olympics and needed a boxing broadcasting team. Frank was tight with Don Ohlmeyer, the reigning network czar, so happily I signed with him and stayed with NBC for 12 wonderful fun-filled years.

CHAPTER 8

My Introduction to NBC

I left Barry Frank's office at IMG, my head in a whirl. I never imagined he was so big and so important, and now he was my agent. While I had been in his office, he had fielded hold-my-hand calls from John Madden and Billie Jean King, who at the time was a tennis superstar.

The optimistic side of me said, "You are in with the big boys! You got it made." Nevertheless, the pessimist in me was whispering, "You are the last guy in line. You'll never get any personal attention from Barry Frank. You're just small potatoes."

✗✗✗✗✗✗

A uniformed guard protected the line of elevators at NBC. I gave my name, and he smiled, welcoming me to the Kingdom of NBC. I felt like a kid on the first day of school. I'd had so many first days, in so many schools, that I was pretty well inured to nervousness. The opposite actually would take place. I got belligerent, expecting the worst, swearing to take no shit. It wasn't a bad way to deal with television executives.

The door opened, and a large, tubby man was waiting to greet me.

"Hiya, Doc!" he said through big, blubbery lips. "I'm Michael I. Cohen. The 'I' stands for 'Ink.' I'm head of publicity around here."

He pumped my hand vigorously. The guy was six feet tall and looked like a rugby player gone to seed. He was sloppy, and there were mustard and ketchup stains on his sweater. His tie was loose, and the rolls of fat under his chin nicely fit in the chasm between each end of his collar. His face was overly large, dominated by a red bulb of a nose, and his piggy blue eyes twinkled when he talked, and he talked all of the time. I loved the guy at first glance.

"Come to my office, Doc. I gotta talk to you," he whispered conspiratorially.

His office was small, made smaller by the clutter. He obviously never used his garbage can; every nook and cranny was filled with old *New York Times* newspapers, magazines, and unopened mail.

"Sit down. I need to brief you before you meet the hoi polloi. I got the lowdown on you from the press guys. They say you're a straight guy, a real stand-up guy who won't take shit from nobody." He grinned and grabbed a half-eaten hot dog, cramming it into his mouth. "This'll be fun! I've been needing an outside guy to watch my back, and you'll be needing an inside guy."

This guy was funny, I thought, and ballsy, too. I really liked that.

"Mr. Inside," I said, sticking out my hand.

"Mr. Outside," Cohen said, grinning, with a mouthful of hot dog.

An effeminate male voice came from outside the door, "Ohlmeyer's waiting for him," he said.

Cohen walked to the door, swung it open, and said, "Go fuck a duck, you faggot," and slammed the door in the man's face. Cohen chuckled. "He's scared shitless of me."

"But Ohlmeyer ..." I said, indicating I had to go.

"Okay. We'll take this up after you see Don. Here is what you got to know. He's a graduate of the ABC Stalinist regime. They believe in yelling, insulting, intimidating, humiliating, and pushing you around. This first meeting is crucial. Walk in there like John Wayne. You don't know who he is. His reputation means nothing to you. You come from the real world, ghetto medicine, and 17 years with the mighty Ali. How can you be impressed by this flabby guy?

"The good part is if he can't badger you, then he's fair. If he trusts you, you've got carte blanche. They're hiring you because he's scared shitless of boxing. That whole crew over at ABC almost went to the penitentiary because they kept putting on phony Don King boxing tournaments, even after they knew it was phony. Alec Wallau saved their ass by doing a great job of uncovering the facts. Jim Spence and Roone Arledge went before Congress, lifted their right arms, and swore they had no knowledge that the tournament was rigged. Don Ohlmeyer had been badly burned and didn't want to be personally responsible."

I already knew all that, because I knew Don King very well.

"Yeah, I heard they gave me a good going over and found no strings. One thing, though, I won't take this job unless my word is final on any deal I make for a fight. If King or Arum can pick up a phone and talk to Ohlmeyer, then I'm useless."

"Well, tell him up front, right now. I told you, he's scared shitless, especially of Don King, and he hates to deal with Arum. That one will be easy," Cohen stated as we walked out the door.

Cohen had now officially adopted me and drafted me for his team. NBC was neatly divided. Half the place worshipped Cohen and half hated him with a passion.

Without knocking, exhibiting that casual familiarity and lack of respect, which alienated so many executives, Cohen sauntered into Ohlmeyer's office. Ohlmeyer was on the phone with an important call (when a TV exec is on the phone, it's always an important call), but he motioned us to sit down. Cohen was impervious to his gentle hints and pushed behind Ohlmeyer to grab a Diet Coke, opening it noisily as Ohlmeyer turned and gave him a dirty look.

Don Ohlmeyer was tall and good-looking in a waspy Notre Dame sort of way. He finished his phone call, stood up, and extended his hand to me.

"Dr. Pacheco. I know you from *Monday Night Football,*" he said, starting out on the right foot, or so I thought.

"Yes, that was in the days when Cosell was my pal," I said.

Ohlmeyer laughed and nodded his head.

"Yeah, that's Howard. He was your greatest booster and admirer until you started calling fights on TV. Then you became the enemy. I wouldn't take it too hard, though; he doesn't like me, either."

We shot the breeze about life in the Ali circus, and I discussed some of the 12 world champions I had worked with. Clearly he was happy to have me, and the meeting was all warm and cheerful. While we talked, Cohen sat back in a corner of the room, smiling like a lynx. Then we got down to the point of the meeting.

"What is it you want from me?" I asked Ohlmeyer, giving him my best tell-me-the-truth stare.

"Well, for right now, we need you to work the fights we have coming up. We're searching for a good partner for you, but your opinion on them will be asked. We'll let that ride for a few months, then if it all clicks, I've got bigger things in mind," he said, giving me a knowing smile.

I stood up, readying for my parting shot. "By the way," I said, "I have very strong opinions about boxing, and they're based on many years of experience. I don't want, nor will I accept, any opinions on boxing from anyone up here, including you. The point of your hiring me is because I know what I'm doing, so I don't want any interference, or I'll walk. Is that understood?"

He nodded, visibly struggling to control his temper, but still ready to shake my hand. "Do you see anything wrong with what we're doing right now?"

He had opened the window, so I flew on in.

"Yes. I'll tell you now, I won't be part of any telecast produced by Harold Smith. He's a fraud, a paperhanger; he's wanted in Texas; and he's a consummate con artist. I don't know about you, but I don't like testifying in court, and he's using you to get credibility, so you're going to do court time, but Smith's going to do jail time."

Smith was a hall of fame con artist in the boxing world. Even "Yellow Kid" Weil, Doc Kearns, and Tex Ricard paled in comparison to him. When I first met him, he was just another hanger-on in the Ali circus. Most of the guys had police records, and nobody paid any attention to it. Smith had forged checks—hung bad paper—all over Texas, but we didn't know that until much later.

"Cohen, take Ferdie down to see Dick [Auerbach]," he said, adding, "I never liked that guy from the beginning."

As we walked away from Ohlmeyer's office, Cohen pounded my back with his beefy hand. He was walking on air.

"Boy, that was great! I never saw Ohlmeyer back out like he did when you put up or shut-upped him. You'll be on top for a while. Now all you have to do is produce great fights for cheap bucks."

"No problema," I said, wondering where I would start to do that and when I'd be called upon to do just that—take over boxing on NBC.

Dick Auerbach was a slick, 50-ish New Yorker who had played the hallway game at NBC and had earned a second-level executive position. At the time he was in charge of boxing, and he knew nothing about it, which somehow in those days qualified him to be put in charge of the operation. Besides he was in cruise control, headed for retirement, and didn't want any trouble of any kind.

Auerbach was of the Frank Sinatra school of New York cool. He was fashionably dressed, chain-smoked long cigarettes, and wore trendy glasses that made him look like an airline pilot. Cohen's lowdown on him told me that he was a two-faced liar and consummate politician, and he couldn't be trusted. I didn't think Auerbach was too happy to have me added to the boxing program.

When we walked in, Auerbach had his $300 loafers propped up on his desk and he was looking out the window at the New York skyline, which was enshrouded in a gray fog. As was usual for all of these TV execs, he was on an important call. Cohen and I sat down, and Auerbach looked at Cohen as if he was looking at a pile of dog poop. Cohen just smiled broadly. He loved to rile up the executives.

As luck would have it, Auerbach was talking on the phone to Harold Smith. Suddenly, without telling Smith, Auerbach did something I detest. He flicked on the speakerphone and then said, "Harold, we've just hired Ferdie Pacheco, The Fight Doctor from Ali's circus. What do you think of him?"

Of course, Smith spewed forth a nonstop line of hatred. Smith knew I was the man that could ruin his connection to NBC, and he would do anything to fight it.

Any way you look at it, in my book that speakerphone stunt was a real low-life move. Auerbach just grinned and clicked it off, barely able to conceal his joy. He told Smith that I was sitting right there in front of him. Smith had just dug his own grave at NBC.

Nothing about Smith tipped you off about his con schemes. He looked normal, which made him stand out in the Ali circus. He was very friendly, very easy to like, and very easy to trust. He was definitely one of the finest liars I have ever come across.

With Smith's connection to Ali, he sought to parlay the alliance into a con game. Soon he found both Ali and Joe Frazier were sponsoring amateur boxing teams. Reaching out to a confederate in Australia, he suggested a tournament between the two amateur boxing teams be fought there. That done, he eased on up to see Auerbach who, being a true network nitwit, saw only the names Ali–Frazier and broke all speed records signing a $600,000 contract for the whole tournament to be broadcast on NBC. The problem was NBC wouldn't pay until the fights were completed. In other words, Smith needed the money up front to start the con. No one asked how, but he got the money. (When I got there, it was the first thing I asked.)

Smith's explanation to Auerbach was so outrageous it was laughable. He explained that sometime after his ancestors were freed from slavery, they began share-cropping in South Carolina, where they remained for several generations until recently, when the old homestead burned down and the only thing left was an old chimney. He said that he had found old Maxwell House coffee cans in the chimney that contained over $600,000, just enough to finance the Australian tournament.

That cockamamie story was good enough for Auerbach to accept. After all, it was an attractive offer and the explanation sounded good to him.

When I came onboard, I patiently explained the scam to Ohlmeyer, that Smith was using the NBC contract to scam an illegal loan from a bank, and we dropped him like a hot potato. Auerbach was not happy.

CHAPTER 9

Ring Deaths

A painful subject for me is death in the ring. It is a sore point, but boxing is not the number-one sport in deaths. Jockeys have that honor. There are eight or more sports every year that are ahead of boxing in sports-related deaths. Boxing even follows behind baseball, football, and golf! Yes, golf. Think of the lightning, flying golf balls, and heart attacks from the tremendous amount of stress some of these people build up just hitting a tiny white ball. Amazing!

So why is a boxing death so prominent? And why does it appear so unnecessary? Let's begin with the most unpalatable fact about boxing; it's meant to hurt. Sure, there's plenty of pain in football, but that isn't football's main purpose. In boxing, the combatants are out to do damage to one another. It's brutal, it's primitive, and in this day and age should probably be banned. But so should bull fighting, car racing, and war.

The 25 years I've been reporting on boxing have also been spent trying to make it a safer sport. Ohlmeyer gave me an open mike to air pieces on boxing safety, and because he did, I believe I made boxing safer. I began by criticizing a referee's performance. Being mentioned on national TV is a serious weapon to wield. In the past, a referee was pretty well black-balled if he stopped a bout too soon. In the brutally tough times of the 1930s and 1940s, the audience expected blood and gore, and even death. If a ref stopped a fight because one fighter was taking a licking, the crowd would boo and pelt him with beer bottles, so refs traditionally let the fight go on until the fighter couldn't.

A classic example was the Jack Dempsey annihilation of big Jess Willard for the heavyweight title in 1919. When the first round was over, Willard had a fracture of the orbital ridge of one eye, a fractured nose, and eight teeth knocked out, and they later discovered his jaw was broken in 16 pieces, and he had three broken ribs. He was dragged to the corner, and the ref still let the fight continue. That would never happen today. Refs came up to me before a fight and asked me not to say anything bad about them, and my reply was always the same.

"Do a good job, protect the fighter, and you'll get nothing but praise from me."

The same worked for cornermen. This part is even harder. The corner man has trained a fighter for weeks to win at all cost. Any hint of the fighter being a quitter, and he is run out of the gym. Many a fight has been won by a boxer who has been taking a fearful licking, but who comes back through the pain and through the blood to knock out his opponent. Just watch all of the *Rocky* movies.

Yes, it is the reality of boxing, but when is it wiser, for the future health of the fighter, to throw in the towel? To save a brave fighter to fight again another day? Down the road of insanely brave boxers lies probable brain damage and blindness. Is any sport worth that? Hell no, I yelled then and kept on yelling on the NBC microphones until cornermen felt justified in stopping a fight gone wild.

Some cornermen, such as wise old Eddie Futch, earned the praise and gratitude of the public when he stopped a blinded Joe Frazier from answering the bell for the 15th round against Ali in Manila. Angelo Dundee stopped Jimmy Ellis from absorbing a big beating from Frazier in the Garden. Cornermen everywhere noticed. It was no disgrace to save the boxer. I applauded them publicly, and I believe I had as much right as any commentator alive (with the exception of Gil Clancy), because I had spent nearly 20 years working in corners and was even more guilty of the crimes the other braver-than-the-fighter cornermen were, because I was a doctor, and a damned dedicated one, but I was seduced by the lure of the primitive combat of boxing. I had that same win-at-any-price philosophy until, at long last, I had an epiphany.

The change started happening to me after the first Ali–Frazier fight. When I examined Ali and saw the fearful damage he had sustained, and then when I found out Frazier had gone to the hospital for six weeks and had almost died, I began to wake up, but I didn't know how to wake anybody else up. Honestly, I didn't know if I should.

Much time went by, and I watched helplessly as Ali's body began falling apart. The worst day of my life was watching the savagery of the Thrilla in Manila. My conscience ached as I saw Frazier and Ali tear at each other like primordial beasts, until the 10th round, when Ali plopped on the stool, his shoulders heaving, sweat pouring off him like a waterfall, and he gasped, "This must be what death is like. I feel like I'm dying."

Finally I couldn't stand seeing him being beaten to pieces anymore. I quit. I gave him chapter and verse about what was ahead for him medically. Ali heard me, Ali understood, but Ali was in the business of being Ali. Headlines and spotlights were his world. He chose to go on, and there was no self-deception. He knew he'd pay the price, and he chose to do so.

Those around him encouraged him shamelessly until we were treated to the humiliation at the hands of his ex-sparring partner, Larry Holmes. Now we see the results; mid-brain damage, advanced Parkinson's. Could it have been avoided? Hell, yes! If Ali had quit after the first Frazier fight, he would have been fine. If he had quit after the savagery of Manila, he would probably have recovered as well. But he went on.

So, as a cornerman, my career had seen its last day. I wanted no part of being the active participant in a boxing match anymore. Had I enjoyed it? Yes, it was a huge high, particularly going to championship nights. Did I miss it? Yes, heaven help me. I miss it to this day. If I had a chance to work on an Ali fight or call it from ringside on TV, it would be a no-brainer. I'd throw on my red sweater, pack the pockets with gauze and cotton pads, antiseptic and smelling salts, and be there in a flash.

My main complaint about TV boxing was the cavalier way they treated death in the ring. Harshness and insensibility come over even the meekest, most Milquetoast of producers and TV executives. It's as if that is not a real human being dying in front of your eyes, as if the poor victim doesn't have a mom and dad, a wife and child. Like this is some kind of electronic game at the mall.

After Ray "Boom Boom" Mancini killed Korean fighter Duc Koo Kim in the ring we began to do a lot of "Boom Boom" fights. Each and every time there would be the full footage of the poor Korean kid being killed. I raised hell. Didn't they have any compassion, any empathy, and for that matter, any conscience? "Boom Boom" was as kind and nice a fighter as ever fought. A network brought Duc Koo Kim's mother to

America, and she promptly swallowed a bottle of lye. I'm sure some executive was cursing his luck that they didn't have the cameras on her when she did it. The bastards just wouldn't leave it be.

Let me tell you about the deaths I personally witnessed in the ring. When I went to work in the corners, I never guessed I'd be part of tragedy, but how wrong I was.

Emile Griffith was a simple, happy island boy with a beautiful smile and an impressive physique. He had a great corner team in Gil Clancy, his manager; Howie Albert; and Sid Martin, both good boxing men. Griffith was what we outside the New York universe called *protected.* Loosely translated, it means Griffith would never lose any close decisions in Madison Square Garden. He didn't need much help, believe me. He was a great welterweight, the middleweight champ.

The press also loved Griffith. Everyone knew Griffith was gay— yes, boxers can be gay—and for publicity's sake they married him off to a buxom blonde. The ordeal was about as convincing as Rock Hudson's marriage. That little tidbit isn't really anyone's business, but it ties in heavily with the death of boxer Benny "Kid" Paret.

The first fight between Paret and Griffith, in April 1961, was very close, but Griffith won by a knockout in the 13th round and lifted the title. Then Paret got a quick New York rematch nearly six months later and won his title back, setting the stage for the third match. By this time there was real bad blood between the two fighters. The chips started falling into place for their fateful 1962 fight.

The weigh-in at the third fight was mayhem. Paret and his Cuban street people began openly jeering Griffith and his mate. The TV covered Paret saying to Griffith's wife, "I'm gonna whip your ass and then beat your husband's ass!" Griffith was seething.

Now came the crucial chip. The appointed referee, Ruby Goldstein, was the best in the business. The problem was that Goldstein had had a serious heart attack and he was not yet fully recovered. He should never have been allowed to officiate that fight in the first place.

The other chip was that Paret had recently boxed a middleweight fight with Gene Fullmer, a Mormon built like a giant Sequoia tree. He was thick and awkward, and he punched hard. He beat the lighter Paret to a pulp. Now, with not enough time elapsing between that fear-inducing beating and this match, Paret was still in tough shape. His brain was ripe to explode.

On March 24, 1962, Griffith, fighting in a rage, got the damaged Paret in a corner and in trouble, and began to rain down punches on him. Goldstein moved in but didn't have the strength to pull Griffith off Paret. Paret was out on his feet, but his right arm was looped over the top rope, and he hung suspended like Christ on the cross as Griffith flailed away and beat the life out of him.

I watched the whole story, and I was sickened by that spectacle. It was the first ring death I had seen, and I went home and prayed I'd never see another, only to find it happening again.

✗✗✗✗✗✗✗

Paret was in the ring that fateful night because of a series of events that had taken place two years before. Boxing was the favorite sport in Havana, and the best welterweight in the world was Cuba's Luis Manuel Rodriguez. He'd beaten Paret twice in the amateurs. Rodriguez's manager was his uncle, a sour cripple who had an intense distrust of Yankees, so he didn't want Rodriguez to fight in the United States.

Don Jordan was an Indian who had a disastrous liking for drugs and firewater. He belonged to Frankie Carbo, a Mafia man who controlled boxing. Jordan ended up beaten out of his title on his very next fight. Carbo offered the title fight up to Rodriguez, with his usual stipulation of 50 percent, but the old man refused and couldn't be budged. He cost Rodriguez four valuable years of waiting before he got into the ring with Griffith. Paret, who already belonged to Carbo, was substituted for Rodriguez and beat Jordan.

That's where I came in. Chris and Angelo Dundee had made a deal to take over all of the Cuban boxers who had fled from Castro, and soon waves of major-league talent washed ashore at the Fifth Street Gym. Along with Rodriguez and Florentino Fernandez, there was an undefeated featherweight named Ultiminio "Sugar" Ramos. Bob Martin, the premier bookie and purveyor of raw talent, told me, "Bet these two kids, Cassius Clay and Ultiminio Sugar Ramos, until they lose, and you'll get rich." How right he was.

We journeyed to Los Angeles for Rodriguez to fight Griffith at Dodger Stadium on March 21, 1963, and Ramos to fight for the featherweight title against the tough champion, the "Springfield Rifle," Davey Moore (not the same Davey Moore who died in the freak car accident). We were, of course, underdogs in both matchups.

Rodriguez handily won 10-5 over a surprised Griffith, no sweat. We changed cornermen sweaters and came out for Ramos. No one had any knowledge of the altercation that had happened between Moore and his jealous wife before the fight.

BLOOD ^{IN} _{MY} COFFEE

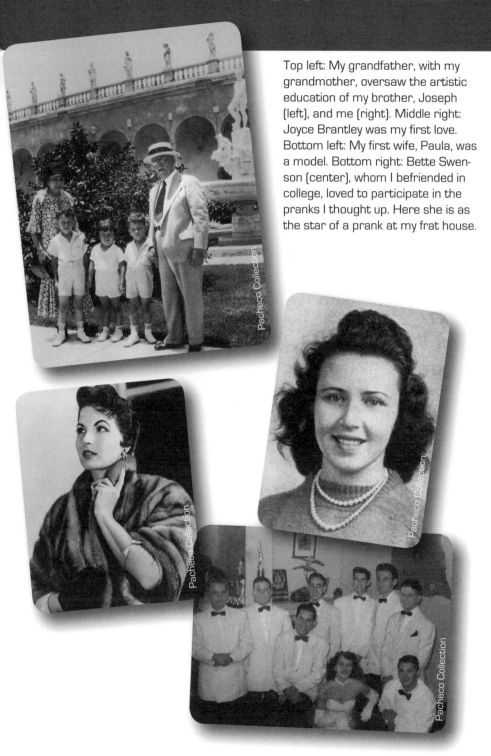

Top left: My grandfather, with my grandmother, oversaw the artistic education of my brother, Joseph (left), and me (right). Middle right: Joyce Brantley was my first love. Bottom left: My first wife, Paula, was a model. Bottom right: Bette Swenson (center), whom I befriended in college, loved to participate in the pranks I thought up. Here she is as the star of a prank at my frat house.

Pacheco Collection

At my office in the Miami ghetto on Second Avenue and 10th Street, I, with the help of my nurse, Mabel Norwood (top right), fulfilled my father's wish that I use my gifts to help those less fortunate. It also provided me access to becoming The Fight Doctor because I ministered to the boxers at the famous Fifth Street Gym.

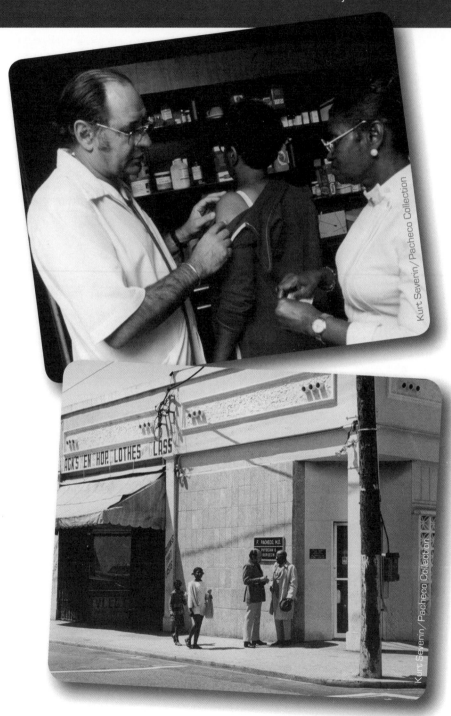

After I began taking care of the boxers' medical needs, I became a cornerman. Top: Angelo Dundee and I work the corner for "Big Al" Jones. Angelo was a master at directing boxers to adjust to their opponents' weaknesses. Bottom: Lou Esa kisses me in gratitude as I tend to him in the ring. Esa was never a boxing big name, but he had a big heart.

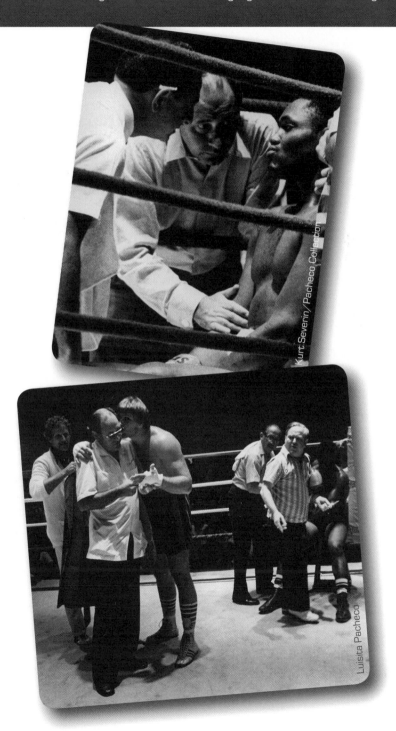

Kurt Severin/Pacheco Collection

Luisita Pacheco

For 17 years I was Muhammad Ali's doctor and friend. Top left: Ali and I stand with our daughters in front of my 1937 Packard limousine. Top right: I stitch up Ali's eye after a fight. Bottom: Ali, Budd Schulberg (far right), and I chat before a fight.

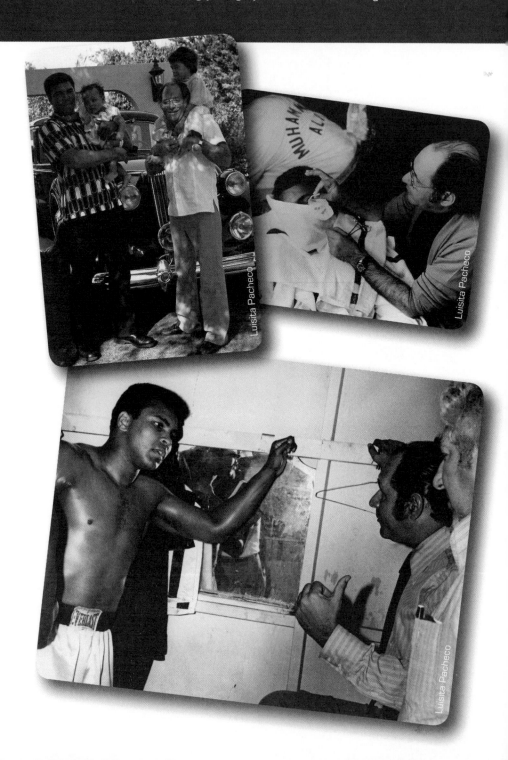

Luisita Pacheco

Luisita Pacheco

Luisita Pacheco

During my time at the Fifth Street Gym, I got to know many of boxing's great characters. Top left: Don King and I stand in front of my burned-out office after the Overtown ghetto riots. Top right: I give some last-minute instructions to James "Great Scott" during the Rahway State Penitentiary fights. Bottom left: I watch a young Roberto Duran train. Bottom right: I helped prolong the life of Budd Schulberg's wife, Geraldine (center), during her bout with cancer.

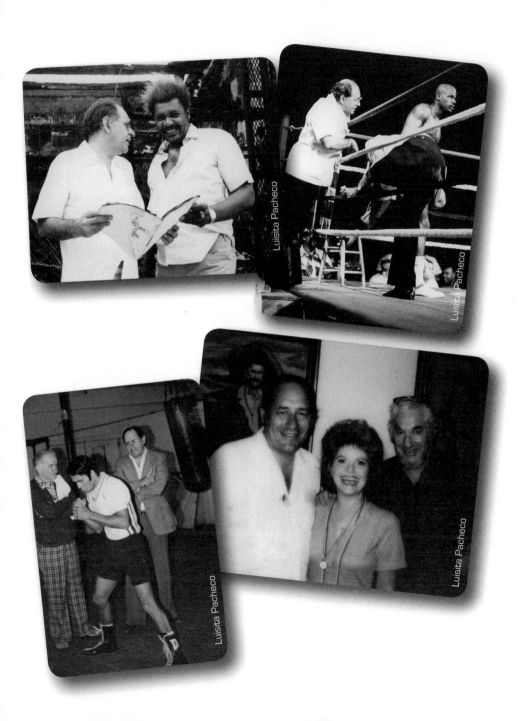

Luisita Pacheco

After I left the corner, I joined NBC to broadcast fights ringside. Top: Brent Musburger pulled me to the mike ringside after he realized he was in over his head. Middle: Producer Mike Weisman gave my partner, Marv Albert (second from left), and me this wonderful welcoming committee when we arrived in Las Vegas. Bottom: Weisman, the TV wunderkind, was the only genius in production I met in my 25 years working fights.

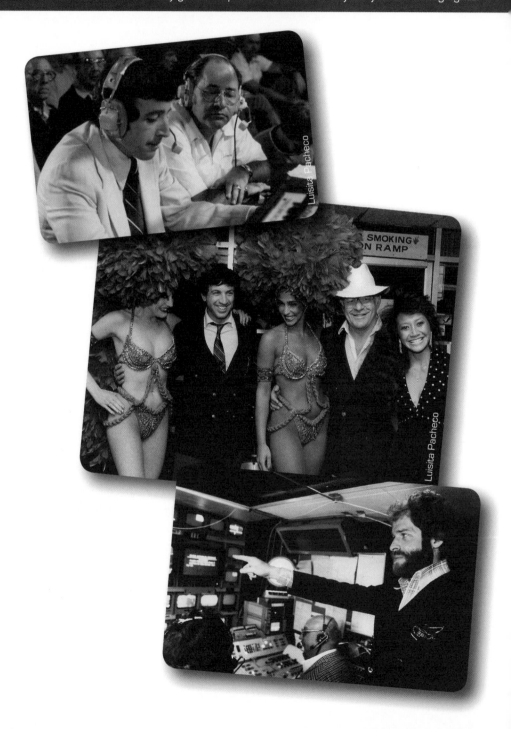

Luisita Pacheco

Luisita Pacheco

Aside from my job as The Fight Doctor and a TV boxing analyst, I was able to express my artistic side through drawing, painting, and writing. The cartoon is one of the sketches from the Seoul Olympics, which caused quite a stir in the Korean press.

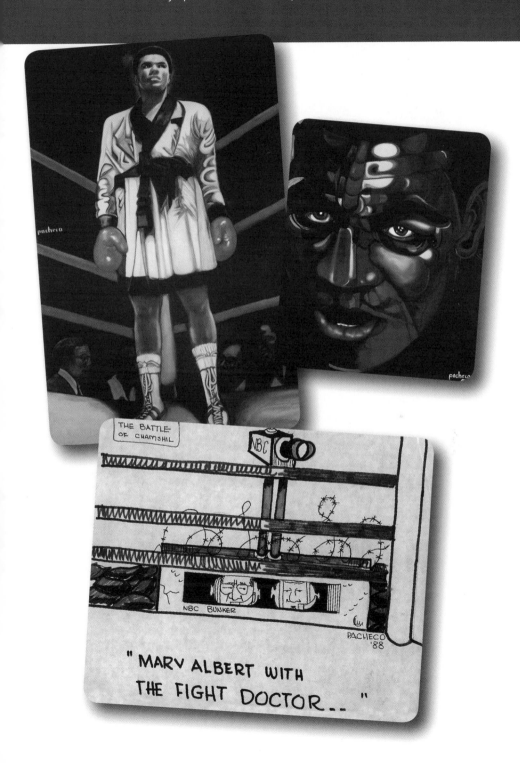

THE BATTLE OF CHAMSHIL

NBC

NBC BUNKER

PACHECO '88

" MARV ALBERT WITH THE FIGHT DOCTOR.. "

Throughout my life, my wife, Luisita, and my daughter, Tina, have been my inspiration and my support. Luisita and I share a lot of things in common. She is an artist—a talented dancer—and a great cook.

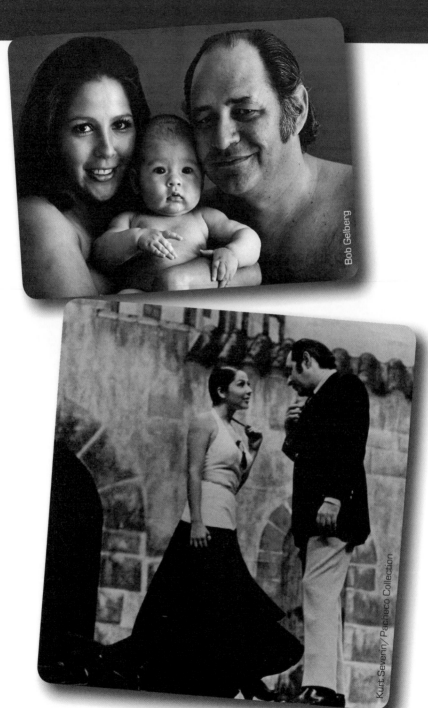

Bob Gelberg

Kurt Severin/Pacheco Collection

The week before, Moore had been speaking at a meeting and hadn't gotten home until midnight. In a jealous rage, thinking the worst of her husband, she had clobbered him on the base of his skull with a Louisville Slugger when he had walked in the door. Down and out he went.

When he came out to fight, he was in horrible shape. No one knew his brain was a ticking time bomb. The fight was brilliant, a real give and take, and it looked like Ramos would get knocked out at any moment. Then, as I was losing all hope, Ramos caught Moore with a devastating combination in the 10th round. His head bounced off the bottom strand of taught rope, and it whiplashed him hard, headfirst on the canvas floor. Moore was counted out, and later, in the dressing room, he said to one of the newsmen, "I got a terrible headache on this side." Then he put his gloved hand on his head and slipped into a coma. Four days later, mercifully, he died.

We had planned to hit the cover of *Sports Illustrated* with a big story on Rodriguez, written by Mort Sharnik. He had spent three weeks with our camp to get the story, and then Moore died suddenly. What a blow! That made me start looking at boxing in a different light.

In boxing, death frequently results because of prior injuries. Alejandro Laverante took a big beating from Cassius Clay, and in Alejandro's next fight, he died. The papers never mentioned that.

CHAPTER 10

Partnerships

At age 50, I was faced with the daunting prospect of having to break in a new partner at NBC. I knew absolutely nothing about broadcasting, but I knew I was a major league talker and had encyclopedic knowledge of my sport, boxing. What I needed was to be paired with a master broadcaster, preferably one who knew nothing about boxing. The choice was not going to be mine. Publicity guru Mike Cohen did his Mr. Inside work and got the genius Mike Weisman to find a partner.

Weisman, who was the only true genius I ran into in 25 years of television, was an easy-going, cool guy who seemed to toss out brilliant ideas as if they were last-minute tidbits. Weisman was a skinny, tall man with reddish hair and a beard. He was one of the few young guys on whom a beard looked good. Later, when he became executive vice president of sports, NBC gave him a clothing allowance, and he appeared in the pages of *GQ*.

Weisman didn't give you the impression that he thought he was the best. He moved with the grace and ease of a man who knew, in his bones, that he was by far the best. As I have observed him for 25 years, I like to say Mike Weisman looks comfortable in his skin. I can't imagine anyone else in there. Only Mike Weisman can be Mike Weisman. He came to work as if he were visiting his frat house. He had been a ballplayer, and he had an athlete's grace of motion.

Nothing seemed to rattle him. Although almost everyone at NBC overreacted to every little thing we did (I called that the sky-is-falling-Chicken-Little psychosis), Weisman laughed and came up with an idea to put out the fire. Weisman was pure television. He had not done radio. He came from a sports-TV-radio family. If this all seems an oddly long way to go to introduce my broadcast partner, Marv Albert, you will see how smart Weisman was in picking Albert and how sharp he was in molding us into a team. No one recognized it was Weisman's subtle and light direction that was responsible for the great boxing team that we became. No one knew. I did.

Marv Albert was a pure star. He was motivated and driven by a desire to be perfect. Once he undertook a job, his employer could be sure Albert would devote 110 percent of his waking hours to be the best he could be, which was, usually, the best in the business. Professionally, his reputation and credentials were impeccable. He had majored in broadcasting at Syracuse, the best university in America for broadcasting, and graduated from NYU. Typically, he excelled.

I'd never heard of him, because Albert was at this time only a New York media star. But he was all over the place. He did the news at WNBC at 6 p.m. and 11 p.m. every night. He did Jets, Rangers, and Knicks games. Miraculously, unless they overlapped, he never missed a game. I watched him do the news, get into a limo, drive to Atlantic City, do a fight, get back into the limo to get back to Newark to do a hockey game, and then do the 11 p.m. news.

Watching Albert in action, I realized I was in the presence of an industrial-strength workaholic. He had no time for anything outside of sports. He had a perfect, beautiful wife named Benita, and three children. He seemed to mold their family life around his career demands. Albert even taught his sons broadcasting by setting up a station in his house. His son, Kenny, is today a successful TV sports broadcaster, thanks to his father working with him.

When Cohen called to tell me that I had to come to New York to go to a Madison Square Garden fight with Weisman and my prospective partner, I was filled with curiosity. As soon as I heard Weisman was involved, I relaxed. I knew he would pick a winner for me, so I approached meeting Albert with high hopes.

Cohen had taken us to one of his many crony-packed smoky sports bars, with Weisman dragging Albert along. Weisman fit in everywhere, while Albert looked out of place. Albert appeared affable enough, but his friendliness did not appear genuine. Try as he might, he looked uncomfortable. Looking back, after I got to know him very well, I could understand his discomfort. After all, here he was a major fixture in media-driven sports, acknowledged as the very best New York had to offer, and he was being called to audition for the role as the blow-by-blow announcer to a doctor who had scant experience in broadcasting fights. If Ohlmeyer and Weisman said Albert was the man, though, so it was. They knew best. We didn't have to like each other. We weren't getting married; we were just doing a show.

From the start I could see Albert did not like fights. I doubt if he had even seen a fight up close. I watched him closely as his face held a look of revulsion with every punch. Distaste was on his face as we were sprayed with sweat and blood, and a look of relief appeared as each round ended. I talked and talked to him through the fights, because I wanted him to be at ease with the thought that I not only knew every aspect of boxing but had a lot of stories of boxing and that I was funny and irreverent. Albert was an easy target, and I certainly did not respect the aura of untouchability he enjoyed on TV. To begin with, I was vastly older than he was, a much better educated man, a doctor, and a man of considerable accomplishments. I had even been awarded a team Emmy for the work on my first show on CBS, the first Ali–Spinks fight with Brent Musburger.

When Albert and I finished that first night at the Garden, I was satisfied that we had found my partner. The more he tried to fend off jibes about his toupee, impossibly square clothes, and absurd neckties, the better the mix would be. At first he looked very uncomfortable when I poked fun at him. But as the public liked our chemistry, he adjusted and came around to the point where he was giving as good as he got. We formed a great comedy team. It took years, but give Albert credit, he got better and better, and in our later years we appeared to be loose and enjoying our hours behind the microphone. For me, it was a very happy time, and I felt fortunate to work next to a guy who was a perfectionist and the best in the business.

From Albert I learned to quit taking the job so lightly. This was specifically true in the pronunciation of proper names. I come from a culture in Ybor City where everyone made fun of people with hard-to-pronounce names. So when a Russian boxer showed up with an unpronounceable name, I found a word that sounded like the Russian's name. "Cheracol, sounds like a cough syrup, drops a straight right hand."

Albert's face dropped in dismay. He had done his homework, and he knew how to pronounce the Russian's name. I laughed at Albert's discomfort and continued to call him Cheracol. Albert was right; I was wrong. It's called professionalism. Albert saved me from professional embarrassment. I ran many games on Albert, which in his seriousness, he never seemed to get the point that I was putting him on.

We were featuring an Olympic fighter named Alex Ramos, from New York. Hispanics pronounced the name *Rah-mos*. Americans called him *Ray-mos*. Albert, seriously involved in getting it right, said, "What is the correct Hispanic pronunciation?"

"Rah-mos," I said with as much of a serious face as I could muster.

"So Rah-mos is what we will be using on the telecast?"

"Right," I assured him.

Then, no sooner did the first round start, I said, "Ray-mos is being hit by a left jab."

Albert almost choked on his coffee, and then I knew I had him. I'd see-saw back and forth between Rah-mos and Ray-mos. Albert was easy to catch.

Albert also never caught on to blood in my coffee.

He was kind of a low-maintenance guy. Once the telecast started, he didn't want distractions. So he ordered and fixed his coffee. Then I started the gag by slapping my forehead.

"Did you feel that? I think it was blood off of Ramos." I'd look at the cup of coffee. "You didn't cover your cup?" I'd say in a very doctoral way something about the threat of blood-related diseases. "You didn't even cover your coffee?"

I checked my head.

That was it. Albert discarded the coffee.

✗✗✗✗✗✗

Albert was a finicky eater. He was keenly aware of pathogenic microbes, and his imagination was active about living animals.

So I waited until he ordered his favorite sports food, a hot dog. Then I made a face so he would see it and say, "What?"

"Do you know what makes up a hot dog? Everything that is not saleable from a pig is thrown into a hot dog. Snout, esophagus, lungs, parts of the pig's feet, its curly tail, internal organs, even its penis."

"Stop, I don't want to hear any more," he groaned, turning a light green.

"Pigs are so dirty that experiments have proven you can feed piglets their own shit and they still grow to be fully grown pigs, which are made into hot dogs."

It got to the point that he hid from me to eat a hot dog. Or if they delivered it to ringside, he said, "Now, Ferdie, shut up. Don't say anything."

Of course I reiterated how filthy the hot dogs were. What made it even funnier is I like hot dogs and ate one or two per fight.

✗✗✗✗✗✗✗

Albert also was standoffish. I made it a point to eat supper with each opposing fighter's camp. It was here that I got all of the good communication for the telecast. Last-minute details, which help before you form your expert opinion of the fight, are discovered at supper, where the fight talk is loose and easy.

Every time I tried to drag Albert to supper with the fighters, he always said, "Aw, no, they just want to talk boxing!"

Well. Yeah. Duh.

I took that in stride and used it to make our team better. Albert didn't know any inside stuff and apparently didn't want to know any. I did. It made me the expert. I knew every side of boxing. That was my job as the boxing expert. Albert was the best at describing the action. He was the best pure blow-by-blow announcer in the business.

✗✗✗✗✗✗✗

When our fight coverage expanded to Europe, I saw another side of Albert.

Albert's fear of microbes was so huge that he packed his own towels, pillowcases, sheets, and other linen. His luggage looked like a wagon train!

Once we were in a quaint seaport resort in Italy. The town of Riva del Garde is ancient and out of the way, and virtually untouched by time. Its only claim to recent fame was that Riva is where Mussolini and Clara Petacci were caught and killed. Aside from that, nothing good came from there. It is a summer resort. Period.

Albert arrived in his own transportation with steamer trunks and assorted bags. He had brought the patient, attractive Benita and the children. In a freezing snowfall he waited on the sidewalk with his bags, patiently stomping his feet to keep warm and waiting for the hotel porter to come and move his vast luggage train in. As fate would have it, the best hotel in town, which was built into the side of a mountain, was closed for the season and had been opened by the couple who ran it. No porter. No bellboys. No room service. No laundry. No nothing.

I would guess it was one of the darkest moments in Albert's life. Poor solve-all-problems Benita had to carry luggage up to the third floor. Elevators were also not working. It was a trip from hell.

But then again, one man's hell is another man's heaven.

It was here that Luisita and I experienced one of those rare beautiful moments that come infrequently in life.

After a weigh-in, with no taxicabs running in town, Luisita and I decided to walk back to our hotel, maybe a mile away. Light fluffy snow was falling. I'd never seen snow as beautiful and light. The streets were deserted. No people, no cars. We might as well have been walking in a deserted town in the 14th century. It was as if our happy life was suspended in this silent blanket of white.

We trudged on, arm and arm, realizing we were sharing a magic moment.

We came to an ancient church. It had not been touched since the 12th century. It was small, primitive, lit by one or two candles at the foot of the Virgin Mary. The light was dim with rays of light coming through simple stained-glass windows, shining like spotlights on the Stations of the Cross.

We knelt in prayer before the altar. We had a lot to pray for, a lot to give thanks for. My life had been blessedly happy and so had Luisita's. We had a strong, wonderful marriage and a shining bonus in our daughter, Tina. We stayed a long time in meditation and prayer. Then we walked back in silence, arms entwined, knowing moments like these are to be savored and remembered.

When I got back, I tried to tell Albert and his wife about the walk through the town. They could not understand why I considered these overseas fights as such an opportunity to experience life and learn of the culture of the places we visited. Boxing travels had furnished me with the knowledge of the world. Whether we went to Europe, Africa, Asia, South America, or Australia, we were given the unusual opportunity to learn about our world and its diverse wonders.

One time a world-traveling Napoleon exhibit, the best collection of Napoleonic relics, appeared right across the street from our hotel in Houston. I was amazed that I could not get one person from our crew to cross the street and experience this once-in-a-lifetime gift from France. Only ring announcer Jimmy Lennon came with me.

Lennon and I saw many wondrous sights. We walked the streets of Dublin, went to James Joyce's house, and had tea. But out of 25 years in sports TV traveling, he was the only one I found interested in how life is in other towns. On the other hand, "The Colonel," Bob Sheridan, who calls the fights for Don King, is an expert on bars and pubs on every continent on the globe.

CHAPTER 11

Howard Cosell:
The Cost of Perfection

Cosell and my future broadcasting partner Marv Albert were a matched set in my mind; an entry, 1 and 1A, like racing thoroughbreds. Both were opinionated, abrasive, Jewish New Yorkers, and both wore awful toupees. I never understood that. Both men clung fiercely to that dead rat piece of artificial hair as if it were necessary for life. Cosell had Ali to bedevil him about pulling it off, but Albert had a big no-no about even mentioning it with the NBC crews, except that I had no such restriction and worried him to death about it.

Both men were dedicated, self-promoting, career-driven egomaniacs, who started their careers in New York. Both men were perfectionists who were wound up tightly in their cocoon of self-importance. Both men had highly distinctive speaking styles, which made them instantly recognizable as soon as they spoke their first sentence. I believe they respected each other, although they were only friendly at a distance.

Cosell was a tall man, stooped over from carrying the weight of his importance on his shoulders. He had graduated law school; thus he had his pretensions of intellectual superiority over lesser-educated athletes. He had passed the Bar, but practiced only for a short spell. Then he bought a tape recorder, began reporting Little League sports on radio, and worked his way into New York radio and then to TV.

Cosell befriended the main man in ABC, Leonard Josephson. As long as Cosell had him in his corner, he could ward off the slings and arrows of ABC executives who were always baying and rapping at his heels. His biggest booster was the genius who had single-handedly invented ABC Sports and carried it to the top. That man was Roone Arledge. He loved Cosell's distinctiveness. He appreciated his audience appeal. He was irreverent. He took unpopular positions, defending Jackie Robinson, Floyd Patterson, and Ali in their fight against racial bigotry in sports. He was brutal in bludgeoning athletes over the head with his vocabulary, belittling them for their lack of communication skills. Only Ali could bring him down with his quick wit, mischievous personality, and his fearless ripping off of Cosell's toupee.

People like Roone Arledge are rare in the land of network nitwits. They have an excellent grasp of what television should be. A list of his innovations and accomplishments would fill the rest of this book, but perhaps his most obvious ingenious move was to create *Monday Night Football*, putting Cosell in with a bland foil, Frank Gifford, and an irreverent Don Meredith as a broadcast team and dropping them in the hands of a whipper-snapper producer, Don Ohlmeyer, and a cracker-jack director, Chet Forte. That may be the best team ever assembled to do a sports show. Contrary to what Cosell claimed, *MNF* was not big because of him.

Not that it was a surprise that Cosell thought that he alone is what made *MNF* such a hot show. A true neurotic personality is one who feels that everything that happens in the world is somehow related to him. Once when we were leaving Caracas after George Foreman had dismantled Ken Norton, Cosell got on a plane to New York with Ali and Joe Louis. The plane blew a tire and careened to the side of the runway and hobbled back to the gate. A visibly shaken Cosell came to where I stood.

"Can you imagine if we crashed? Killed in a plane crash with Ali and Joe Louis? Why, I'd be back on page 12 in *The New York Times.*"

He had escaped dying, and his main concern was billing in the obit page. Now *that* is a true neurotic.

One day in Canada he was invited to have lunch with the Canadian Prime Minister Pierre Trudeau. I was standing in the lobby, and he said, "Come on, I've been invited to lunch with Trudeau. I'll take you." In those days we were buddy-buddy because of an involvement with Ali and because in me he saw a fellow—well, in honor of Cosell, I'll say—sesquipedalian.

An intimate lunch with Trudeau? A chance to meet his lovely, wacky wife? Sounded good to me!

We arrived and were ushered into lunch with about 2,000 other people. It was just a political lunch. We weren't within spitting distance of Trudeau. Undaunted, Cosell stomped out. That night, on *Monday Night Football*, Cosell started: "Today I had lunch with Trudeau and he confided in me ..." Cosell proceeded to paraphrase parts of Trudeau's speech.

Next time I saw Cosell, I told him a tale. A Mexican stopped by a stream to water his horse. Suddenly he was aware of a huge *guerillero* behind him on a big black horse. He recognized the man as Pancho Villa. Meekly he saluted the killer. At the same time, the man's horse passed a stool. Villa signaled with his gun that the man should eat his horse's stool. Knowing he would die if he doesn't, the man did so. Villa took the man's horse and rode off. Later that night he was at the cantina trying to drown the taste in his mouth with tequila. The conversation got around to whom was the fiercest bandit, Villa or Zapata. The man said Villa, and moreover, he was a personal friend of Villa's.

"You know Pancho Villa?" the man asked.

"Know him? Hell, I just had lunch with him today."

"You had lunch with Trudeau, huh?" I said.

Cosell walked his rat to the elevator and disappeared.

✗✗✗✗✗✗✗

Both Marv and Howard had perfect wives. They understood that their only rivals would be their husbands' careers, for now at least.

As rotten as Cosell was as an individual, Emmy was good. She understood him, his need to be up front, the center of attention, and she put up with all of his faults, from anti-Semitism to the verbal sexual harassment of any pretty girl within his long reach. Not that he ever cheated on Emmy. He loved himself as only an egomaniac can, but he loved Emmy more. And why not? She was tall and beautiful, bright, brainy, decent, and had no discernable character flaws. She followed the abrasive Cosell, mending fences. She almost succeeded in making him a nice man.

Once, during the time that he considered me his personal enemy just because I had forsaken medicine for a life on TV, I went to the Friar's Club to have supper with my daughter, Tina, who was then just finishing film school at New York University. One good thing about NBC is I got to see Tina regularly when I was in New York.

Across the room I saw Cosell and Emmy having a quiet supper. I had heard Emmy was having a tough time with cancer, and I, along with everyone who knew her, was broken hearted. I walked over, determined not to let Cosell's surly attitude dissuade me from offering a few words of concern and encouragement.

I had my say, studiously avoiding Cosell, and Emmy asked about Tina. They had known her as an infant. When I told her she was at the table, she said they'd pass by on the way out.

I don't know what Emmy said to Cosell, but he was the soul of gentility, wittily conversing with Tina, offering to help her, and in general, being charming. In passing he was even courteous to me. That was the effect Emmy had on him.

Sadly, she died of that affliction, and Cosell was left alone, adrift in a sea of hostility. Cosell's end was not nice. He had alienated almost everyone he had worked with. There was a long list of people in line to kick him when he was down. To his amazement, he found he was unemployable. That, I think was the final blow. When someone who was so studiously revolting finally gets his, it is hard to feel sorrow for him. He was so arrogant, so spiteful, so mean, that his end does not elicit sorrow, just relief.

Like Albert, Cosell worked ceaselessly for perfection. Albert finally blew a safety valve; Cosell just perfected himself away.

The first 10 years of my friendship with Cosell were golden. Because I offered a conduit into the inner circle of Ali, I was his buddy. Ali played with him. Ali was adorable, a little kid making fun of his teacher. Cosell took all of the jiving and loved it, because he got to share the spotlight. Later, he had the nerve to say that he made Ali. Ha! Ali is the sun; Cosell is a dim bulb in his shadow.

He worked fights in a very intelligent way. No one has ever called him dumb or lazy. He did his homework. Before a fight he would always call Angelo Dundee, or Gil Clancy, or Eddie Futch, or whoever managed the corners and ask what to expect. He would hear a full game plan, what to look for, and then Cosell would pass on the information as if it were his own.

I was very friendly with him at this time, because I considered him the best at what he did, and because of his courageous stand on Ali's behalf. Whenever possible, I would pass on inside information that would give him a better picture of the boxers. All of us felt it would make the telecast more entertaining and informative.

One particular day, I was to be treated to the "new" Cosell. The fun-loving, eager-to-work Cosell. The inventive, original, enthusiastic man was replaced by a dour, affected, weary man.

Ali sat on his ring chair and started his usual hour-long press conference. Newsmen appeared from all over the world when he fought, and he was always cordial to one and all, staying as much as one hour after workouts to answer questions. His answers were always colorful, funny, and eminently printable. Ali was on one of his usual rolls. He had seen Cosell, but had not acknowledged him, a slight that rankled Cosell.

"Look at that pathetic spectacle," Cosell said in his new, bored, I've-seen-and-done-everything, weary New Yorker voice. "The guy doesn't know when to get off stage."

He waved a hand in the direction of Ali, who didn't see him.

"The man is a buffoon. A clown. I'm tired of all this childishness."

Frank Gifford, who was with Cosell that day, looked at Cosell in amazement.

"I'm too big for this kooky shit. I don't know why I waste myself with jocks and this child's play," Cosell said. Then he put his arm around me. "You got the right answer. You work in the real world. You're out there in the ghetto, treating those poor blacks and helping the Cubans." He went on in this vein for a while until he got to his point. "I really feel I've done it all. I should be doing something more significant in my life." He looked with glazed eyes at Ali, still babbling away on the ring apron. "Run for the Senate, perhaps."

Gifford and I looked at each other and smiled.

"The United States Senate?" I ventured tentatively.

"Sure, why not? I'm a lawyer, an activist, a famous listened-to voice in America. Look what I did for Robinson, for Patterson, for Ali."

He rose to leave, and Ali saw him and went into his Cosell impersonation, which by this time was pretty good.

"I don't need this," Cosell said, waving his arms and smiling his lynx smile. "The adulation, the recognition, the fame. There, it's all there for the kid. I don't need it. I'm tired of this phony life of sports. It's so infantile."

So saying, the future senator from the State of New York took his body over to where Ali was and did 10 minutes of mugging and gagging around with him. Then he stayed a few minutes signing autographs.

"You think he means it?" Gifford asked me.

"Don't worry. You'll have to kill him to get him off *Monday Night Football*."

Ohlmeyer once told me, "Show me a guy who does not have an ego, who is in front of the cameras, and I'll show you a failure."

In Ohlmeyer's case, and many other gifted artists behind the camera, the same holds true. You need a robust ego to walk the high wire without a net every weekend. Cosell never had that problem. In his mind he was the only performer in television who could do a fight, a baseball or football game, or a horse race. If it was sports, Cosell could do it better than anyone in the world. So saith Cosell.

With an inflated ego came disagreeable, petulant behavior toward his co-workers. Where he was a drooling sycophant around politicos, or A-list celebrities, he was a bully to his co-workers. No longer would he help production persons who needed encouragement or help, but more often than not, he came down hard on them, causing repeated wounds.

He became self-serving and over-inflated his importance beyond recognition, and where before his humor had a funny edge, it now became hard, biting, cutting, and insulting. He was no one you would care to have supper with.

✗✗✗✗✗✗

Where to put Cosell? An aberration? A force of change? A small man thrust in a big role? I think he did make a difference. He opened the ways for big-mouth guys like me, Al McGuire, John Madden, etc., to express our thoughts without worrying about a censor.

Did he know boxing? No. Did he know how to telecast boxing? Yes, because he had a sense of drama. He brought the fans into the fight. He didn't care for Xs and Os; he cared for the feeling of the event, the ebb and flow that is so necessary to follow. I liked to hear him in boxing, but when he loved a fighter, like Sugar Ray Leonard, the call was lopsided and pitifully unfair. His pretension concerning his intellectuality was funny to any educated person. If he was so far above the woeful creature that toils in sports, if he were so much more intelligent and had a bigger social conscience, then why the hell didn't he resign and run for political office? Abandon the low road of sports and elevate himself to the high road of politics?

Because he was an intellectual fraud and he knew it. All puff, and not a deep thought in his toupee.

When Cosell lost Emmy, he lost his will to live. He was alone in a hostile world, without work, without a public. Not even Ali could save him, so he did the only thing he could do—he died.

CHAPTER 12

Africa and Advancement

Auerbach was on the phone with me, all smarmy voiced, "Guess where we're going with the Tate–Coetzee fight?"

"Not South Africa?" I said, kidding on the square.

Even an NBC nitwit couldn't be that stupid. Even in 1979, South Africa was the next thing to Nazi Germany. The repression of blacks had been going on for over a century. They had just had riots in Soweto. Our newsreels were filled with graphic footage showing black-shirted policemen beating up poor black civilians with rubber truncheons. Even more sickening was watching killer police dogs tear at the women and children, who were running away to protect themselves.

There was a long silence as Auerbach tried to figure out why I would be horrified to go to South Africa.

"Ah—yes, Johannesburg. Is there anything wrong with that?"

"Anything?" I was floored. "Everything!"

I launched into a 10-minute tirade on the mess we were dropping NBC Sports into. I hadn't learned one big fact—network sports execs don't live on this earth with all of its problems, they live in a world of their own, and in that world nothing matters except the event.

Here's a good example: Do you remember the NFL playing disgraceful games during the time the nation was mourning the assassination of President John F. Kennedy? There was no TV the day the Japanese bombed Pearl Harbor, but I'll bet if there had been, some network would have covered a football game on that fateful Sunday.

Networks have no conscience, no sense of social awareness. All they see is *the event,* or *the game.*

If you understand that premise, then you can also understand Auerbach's blind acceptance of going to South Africa, where segregation was a fact and racial discrimination a way of life. And here we were, taking a black man there to fight a white man. What's more is that the black man, John Tate, was the Heavyweight Champion of the World, who figured to beat the bejesus out of the white kid, Gerrie Coetzee, who was a big favorite in all of South Africa.

Coetzee was nicknamed "The Bionic Fist," because he had a series of screws and hardware holding his punching hand together. In the history of boxing, there have always been fighters with gimmick punches. In the era of Joe Louis, one of his opponents, Lou Nova, had a punch that he called "The Cosmic Punch." Nova said he had an astrologer figure the curvature of the earth at each location, and if he threw his right hand along that arc, his punch knocked out anybody. Louis was a simple, uneducated black man from Detroit, and his take on Nova was, "I got an 'Earth Punch.'" He said it without smiling, and he knocked Nova out before he had a chance to find his arc. That was the end of "The Cosmic Punch."

Roberto Duran, the fierce Panamanian champion, was called *Manos de Piedra,* "Hands of Stone," and they indeed were. But Coetzee just had a bum hand. Forget the Bionic stuff, Tate was going to knock him out.

Auerbach insisted, "NBC is going to score a first with this fight! It'll be the first time a stadium is going to be desegregated in South Africa. That's certainly a justification for NBC to take its cameras down there."

"Where were you during World War II? Did you sleep through it?" I couldn't believe what I was hearing. "Man, these Dutch guys in South Africa are Nazis. Instead of killing Jews, they're picking on blacks. And, you see, Dick, that is borderline bad because Africa *is* black. The blacks belong in Africa; the whites do not. Are you beginning to feel how offensive this whole fiasco is to all of the blacks in Africa, to say nothing of our own blacks here in America?"

I was getting downright distraught.

"I'm sure it will all work out," he said.

I could see the suave, mindless Auerbach flicking an ash from his long Benson & Hedges, his mind deflecting flimsy afterthoughts. And then it came.

"It's a game, Ferdie. Somebody's got to do the show. We've got to play the game."

✗✗✗✗✗✗

There was a very wealthy South African man named Sol Kurshner, who controlled the big diamond mines and most of the real estate in sight. He was short, but handsome, in his late 30s. But he looked a lot taller when Miss Universe was on his arm. He had everything in the world a playboy could want, and he was, of course, an industrial-strength egomaniac, but who wouldn't be? The man was on top of the world.

So, with a South African kid wanting the world championship so badly, Kurshner decided to buy a chance at it. The one problem was he knew nothing at all about boxing, so he decided to do what he always did when confronted with a problem: He bought what he needed. In this case, a promoter. There were only two in Kurshner's class. One was Don King, an ex-convict, aggressive, and very sassy. The other was a knife-sharp Jewish New York lawyer by the name of Bob Arum, who had risen to fame with Bobby Kennedy. Kurshner was a Jew, too, so the pick was a no-brainer. Arum was his man. He easily divested any semblance of morality or principle—that is if any lawyers have those qualities—and jumped feet first into the immoral morass of big-time boxing.

As to the storm troopers and their dogs, Arum shrugged them off with an easy rationalization, "That was yesterday. Today, all is okay."

I'd been there when Arum got his start in boxing, first as Ali's lawyer and then as his promoter. I liked him. When he's not raping you out of every cent you have, he's nice as he can be. And he's a lot of fun. Besides, I like snakes. He brought lying up to a fine art that only Harold Smith and Don King could match. But, hell, that was boxing.

One last thing came up before we packed our expeditionary force and started out for Africa, and it was a beauty! Don Ohlmeyer is a loyal guy. He doesn't forget people who helped him on the way up. So, while he was on watch, he hired a stepson of the legendary Jim McKay, an ABC star who had helped Ohlmeyer up the ladder. The problem was, this kid, Sean, showed up fresh from Duke University, looking like he was all of 14 years old. His suit looked like he bought it out of the children's department at Macy's. All he needed was a tin lunch pail. Even his hair was cut like a little boy's with one lock falling over his forehead. Granted, he was as nice as he could be, but he was in way over his head in a man's world.

Ohlmeyer didn't know what else to do with Sean, so he made him an executive. Eventually, this little snit was put in charge of me! Talk about a mismatch. Later, when Ohlmeyer left NBC, the kid was shot out of the 16th floor cannon like a Flying Zucchini Brother. He landed in Barry Frank's office and later, when Frank was busy in Yugoslavia, Sean became my manager! See the connection? Please don't laugh. I give little Sean all of the credit in the world. I'm his biggest fan, because Sean McManus is now the president of CBS Sports. El Presidente! Go figure. And he still looks like a teenager. He even got married, maybe just to prove he was of age and could vote.

Ohlmeyer's sense of payback was at play with Africa, also. His biggest booster at ABC had been Howard Cosell. Cosell had a daughter named Hillary, who was as bright as she could be but had inherited her father's annoying superciliousness, his superior attitude, and the unfortunate propensity to patronize everyone around her.

Scratching his head to create a job for Hillary, Ohlmeyer decided to let her do a 10-minute documentary on South Africa. What could he have been thinking? Hillary hated everything about the assignment and ended up turning out a masterpiece of hatred and disgust for the country and its people. Looking at the reel, I was overcome by its brilliance, even if it was entirely opposite of what had been expected. Hillary had her old man's talent of going for the jugular, and she ripped the heart out of the South African government. If we were getting ready to invade, this would have been the piece that would kick off the attack.

Stunned, I stumbled out of the viewing room and was met by a smiling Auerbach.

"Great, huh? Dynamite kid, eh?"

He was practically jumping for joy. I looked at him as if he had lost his mind or found his sense of humor.

"What in hell are you going to do with that incendiary 10 minutes of film?"

"Play it, right before the fight."

"Not in South Africa, you're not." I was adamant. "They'll kill you and disembowel Hillary."

"Well, that gets NBC off the scheme, don't you see? 'Yeah, we're telecasting from there, but we know the place is rotten and we aren't afraid to say it.'"

He smiled in anticipation of the good press he was sure to get in New York.

"Don't give up your passport to anyone and be ready for a precipitous exit," I said, before heading back to the St. Regis Hotel to down a few drinks and try to forget that God made people like Auerbach, Arum, Kurshner, and Hillary Cosell.

Luckily, someone at NBC, who had a sense of survival, had second thoughts about the Cosell piece. So Auerbach said, "Hold off. Let's see what we can do with this."

Arum sat for five minutes in stunned silence as he viewed the dogs attacking women and children. Finally he couldn't take it anymore and yelled, "Are you fucking nuts?" Abandoning any pretense of brother-hood and reverting to the viper he really was. "If you even try to show that, I'll have you arrested. Deported! If NBC shows that, heads are gonna roll." He was livid. "I can't believe this, it's insane! You are guests of South Africa and Sol Kurshner. Do you think for one fucking minute they are going to let that air?"

Auerbach tried to take a reasonable position as an NBC executive, as an American, as a Jew, and finally as a man, but Arum swallowed him whole, like all good snakes do.

Punches were thrown; glasses knocked off. I hustled a badly shaken Auerbach into our car. It was the most hilarious thing I had ever seen, watching two executives fist fight, and pretty poorly at that. I guess they never paid attention to their own sport.

That night we were invited to a first-class soiree at Kurshner's opulent home, which was a veritable palace, located about 35 miles out of town. It was a rainy night, and Auerbach had shown up looking like Humphrey Bogart in *Casablanca*. His trench coat was freshly pressed, and he sported a snap-brimmed, dark brown hat and his ever-present cigarette. In the limousine on the way there I spent my time convincing Auerbach to cool down and show NBC's finest colors.

"And for God's sake, don't mention that awful tape," I cautioned just before the driver let us out and headed back to get another load of NBC clods.

We made a grand, star-quality entrance. The room was packed, and everyone was eating and drinking like it was their only meal in days. Not a soul had noticed us.

"Let's circulate and work the room," I said, heading off in the direction of Miss Universe, who was standing in a circle of admirers.

Auerbach went the opposite direction, which was to his misfortune, because he ran right into Arum, who was still sizzling from their afternoon encounter. I could hear their voices rising, and then Auerbach appeared by my side.

"I'm not staying anyplace that snake is standing," Auerbach declared loudly.

I flashed a mental picture of a snake in a tuxedo, standing straight up, and nearly laughed in his face. Auerbach grabbed his Bogart trench coat, wrestled himself into it, clapped the snappy hat on, and plunged out the door into the rainy night. It was such a great exit, the guests, who had fallen silent during the loud exchange, nearly broke into applause.

Then the front door slowly opened and in came Auerbach, drenched like a drowned Casablanca rat, and whimpering, "Anybody got a ride back to town?"

No one did, and by this time the entire room had heard of the infamous tape and Auerbach was as welcome as Joseph Goebbels. Unfortunately, he had to hang around until his taxi came and had to dole out about $150 for the ride back.

xxxxxx

The stadium sat about 83,000 fans, and there wasn't an empty seat in the place. Albert and I were seated ringside, ankle deep in mud. Behind us, Roberto Duran was yelling his own commentary at me, which he kept up during the entire fight. I think more people heard Duran's call of the fight than mine, and his was in Spanish!

Weisman came out to look at the huge crowd. His experienced eye was looking at what our cameras would show.

"There are 83,000 people here all right. Eighty-two-five are white, and about 500 are black, and sitting on the rim of the stadium. Some integration, huh?" he said to me.

"Maybe you can put Hillary up there with the blacks to make a statement," I said helpfully.

Weisman, great producer that he was, had spotted a bigger problem. The audience was not lit. Only the ring had bright TV lights trained on it, and back in the United States, the audience would think the fight was being held in an empty basement, but it was too late to do anything about it.

"Marv," he said, "I want you to keep repeating every round how many people are here for the fight. Just keep talking about the noise."

"What noise?" Marv said, noticing that most South African fans were courteously sitting on their hands, waiting for the fight to start.

"We'll mike Duran," I interjected. "He's so excited he sounds like 83,000 fans."

"Eighty-three thousand Panamanian fans," Albert said ruefully.

The audience might have been very well behaved, but they were heavily armed as well. It seemed like the South Africans didn't go anywhere without their hunting rifles on the off chance a rogue elephant might charge them, even in a stadium.

At the end of each aisle was a black-uniformed storm trooper holding a rifle, with a large German shepherd dog leashed at his sides. It was quite an intimidating sight.

The fight began. Our ace camera crew jumped on the platforms at each corner of the ring. These were our closeup cameras, a staple at every fight. At the end of round one, a uniformed officer came over and handed me a folded note that read very simply, "If that bloke with the TV camera gets up in the ring again and blocks our view, I'm going to blow his head off."

I quickly called Weisman, who then, with Auerbach trailing behind, cornered Arnie Rief, our short-tempered equipment manager, in the remote viewing truck. Rief was already boiling mad over Auerbach's insinuation that the audience lighting problem was somehow his fault.

He responded in his typical New York way, "Fuck them. I'm not taking my guy down."

Even for an old New Yorker, he was pushing his luck.

"Yes, you are!" Dick bristled, going nose to nose with the enraged Rief. "Fuck them, fuck you, and fuck this truck!" he roared in Rief's face, whereupon the two seemingly mature executives started their own fight.

They locked arms and spilled out of the truck, onto the muddy field, taking Weisman, who was trying to break up the brawl, with them. Looks like the cameras were in the wrong place after all.

Somehow we got through the night. "The Bionic Fist" never landed, but the bionic jaw crumbled under a pile-driving right-hand hook from John Tate. It wasn't nearly as good as what the audience didn't see.

✗✗✗✗✗✗

The result of the Africa fight was that I replaced Auerbach. I was left with the job of making the fights, pricing them, negotiating the contracts, and then calling the fights on TV.

Ohlmeyer was the ideal boss. He grumbled from time to time, but when he was proven wrong, he admitted it and shut up thereafter. A real man there.

Once, we had a fight made with the TV-attractive boxer Sean O'Grady. Our opponent fell out, and there was virtually no time to replace him. However, my boxing sources came up with a tough kid, Andrew Ganigan, who trained in Hawaii.

Ohlmeyer uncharacteristically blew up. He called me up, raging, yelling how could I do that? He lived in Hawaii, and he knew this Ganigan was a bum.

Keeping my temper, I said, "Don, you don't know a fucking thing about boxing. This is going to be a great fight."

"It better be," he said, threateningly.

I just laughed and hung up.

The fight turned out to be all it was billed to be and more. And because O'Grady had a history of being cut, there was blood and gore all over the place. Just what the crowd roared for. Finally, O'Grady won out over Ganigan, but it was mighty close.

When I got back to my room, the phone was ringing. Surprise! It was Ohlmeyer.

"Ferdie, you were right. That's the last time I'll ever second-guess you."

He hung up, and I never heard from him directly again. He was my kind of guy.

✗✗✗✗✗✗

My fights had taken off, and the ratings were high. I was getting great fights at bargain prices, using common sense. Prior to me, network nitwits, not knowing fighters or fight people, depended on Arum and King, fellow New Yorkers, to tie up all dates. It was a lazy and stupid thing to do, because we became the soldiers in their game of Monopoly, and the networks were the cudgels that King and Arum used to preserve his powerful hold.

"If you want to get your boy on TV, then you gotta come through me," I understand King had told ABC, and they obeyed, until he almost got them all thrown in jail. Arum had CBS using Gil Clancey and Mort Sharnick as his inside men. NBC had Dick "Sell Me Anything" Auerbach. Independent promoters were out in the cold; their boxers were jumping ship and fleeing into the waiting arms of King and Arum.

When the word came down that I was the man at NBC, King and Arum each called, saying the same thing, "Now we're in! I can fill up the year for you with great fights!"

Boy, were they in for a surprise!

Patiently I explained that there was no we. This had to do with me, and my allegiance was totally with NBC. However, I proposed to open the doors to all promoters, big or small, whether in New York or Podunk.

Great was their consternation therein, and after much gnashing of the teeth, both sides declared me a traitor. The little promoters could barely believe their good luck. And this was my business ploy—simple as it sounded, it worked.

However, I knew King and Arum would immediately make an end run around me and charge into Ohlmeyer's office. True to his word, Ohlmeyer wouldn't see them. They even tried to get through to the president of NBC, Arthur Watson, and he stood up to them as well. That was it. King and Arum were *persona non grata* at 30 Rockefeller Center.

And so it worked. I'd get a good, solid boxing promoter with years of experience promoting good fights, say maybe Russell Peltz of Philly's Blue Grotto. I'd pick his two best middleweights, both ranked in the top 10 contenders, and I'd say, "I'll only pay $35,000." (A regular TV fight went for between $50,000 and $75,000. If it was King, it was always over $150,000, usually for stiff build-up-his-fighter bouts.)

Peltz was a top boxing brain, but he loved to whine and wheedle and cry. I waited out the crying storm, and then said calmly, "Russell, it's $35,000, but whoever wins comes back on and stays on while he wins, all of the way to the title, and you have an open door at NBC as long as I'm here. And one more thing. If the guy that loses gives me a sensational fight, he'll come back, too. Thirty-five thousand, Russell. See you at the fight."

Peltz, along with Butch Lewis, the Duvas, Murad Muhammad, Phil Alessi, the Dundees, and Mickey Duff (in London, England) came into my NBC stable. The fights were so good and meant so much that I coined the phrase, "Cross Road Fights," which Mike Cohen took to the press.

NBC Cross Road Fights generated great ratings for cheap bucks, and King and Arum worked hard to but never broke up any of the matches with their wily ways. Arum was particularly vicious in his tactics, but he was so open about it that he drew my ire and just kept shooting himself in the foot. King was his old, intimidating gangster self, threatening me with physical violence or threatening to sue NBC for "me-ions," as he would say. But King didn't get where he was by staying mad. He would offer a bribe in an off-handed way or offer a fabulous perk, maintaining a sort of friendly enmity with me. I honestly liked King's personality, his ebullience, and bigger-than-life persona. I always thought his story would make a great Broadway musical, but Paul Robison beat me to it, with *Emperor Jones*.

Ohlmeyer backed me up all the way during my successful run of boxing at NBC against the outrageous slings and arrows of King and Arum. He made it easy for me to implement my open-door policy for promoters.

Shortly after the *Cross Road Fights* series ended, Ohlmeyer tired of his role as Emperor of the World and passed his crown to Weisman. But I can't leave Ohlmeyer without saying something about his human side.

During the time I was at the top of my form, I got a call from a favored promoter who offered me dibs on an unbelievable attraction. Undefeated Sugar Ray Leonard against the champion, "Hands of Stone" Roberto Duran. This was the fight of the decade—red hot. The price? A cool million—a real steal. I was so excited I jumped on a plane to go see Ohlmeyer in person.

But Ohlmeyer didn't react as I anticipated. He had a better fight. He said Muhammad Ali was coming out of retirement for a million. In any network executive's empty mind, an illusory Ali fight was better than Leonard in a real fight with Duran.

I was shocked. I was still involved with Ali. He trained in Miami, where I lived. Or rather, I should say, he *didn't* train. He had no intention of coming back but was having his usual fun with the media. Ohlmeyer, who shouldn't have even taken the call to begin with, took the bait like Harry the Tuna. The name *Ali* was still magic.

When I came in, straight from the airport, bristling with arguments and reasons to snap up the very real Leonard–Duran offer, Ohlmeyer glad-handed me and walked out the door, motioning over his shoulder for me to follow him. I assumed we were taking this decision to Arthur Watson.

As we walked past desk after desk, he motioned for the good-looking girls to follow us. Soon we—suave Ohlmeyer; me, with smoke coming out of my ears; and six twittering, leggy secretaries—were standing at the elevator door. I couldn't get him to discuss what I had come all the way from Miami for. We went to the lobby kiosk, where he bought a Snickers bar for each dimpled beauty. I exploded.

"Did I come all this way just to watch you buy your harem candy bars?" I roared. "Listen, Don, you gotta make a decision or we're going to lose the fight of the year. A million is cheap. It'll go for much more. Ali is not fighting again, so quit jerking off on his mirage. It ain't gonna happen!"

His quick temper got the better of him and he came out with this classic Ohlmeyerism: "You don't understand. You don't have the inalienable right to speak to me like that!"

"Inalienable right?" I choked back a laugh. So now I'm talking to Thomas Jefferson. I turned around with a hasty "Fuck you," and headed straight back to the airport.

We lost the wonderful Leonard fight with Duran (Leonard lost), Ali did not come out of retirement (of course), and NBC missed out. I hope the six Snickers bars paid off.

✗✗✗✗✗✗✗

Linda Johnson, Ohlmeyer's secretary and one of his close and personal friends, found herself in charge of *Sportsworld,* our showcase weekend show.

She didn't like boxing and didn't know anything about fights, but she was very astute, and knew boxing was a ratings winner. I found her very easy to work with.

She had a strange staff, though. As her personal secretary, she had a girl that looked like she was working on a doctorate in medieval mythology. She was a lump, with the personality of someone who spends weeks on end in libraries and takes vacations alone to Siberia.

Johnson's other assistant was the much-maligned Matthew McCarthy, who eventually succumbed to a hard right-hand punch to the teeth by the bull-like macho man Mike I. Cohen. Regrettably, that brought about Cohen's demise. McCarthy belonged in sports like I belong in a luge run. He wore lovely pastel sweaters, blow-dried his wavy hair, and, some swear, wore makeup. I never noticed any makeup on McCarthy. Well, maybe a little blush. What he was doing in the manly world of TV sports, I could never guess. He could talk for hours about poetry and theater, but he had no clue who Roberto Duran was, much less Tony Zale or Rocky Graziano. Yet, he had the producer's ear.

So I learned that the way to treat a setup like that was to create a sort of vacuum between them and me, which I had by living in Miami. But, I ran afoul of the lovely producer, and it was painful for both of us, because we were both in the wrong.

NBC was airing an ill-advised attempt to feature the boxers who should have been going to the Moscow Olympics—which President Jimmy Carter boycotted for the United States. Some of them were good, but most were nothing to write home about, and a few were just plain awful. Any way you look at it, they just weren't professional boxers.

We took a load of them to Lake Tahoe to feature them in a series of bouts. One fight was a legitimate barnburner between a tough Irish New York street fighter, Kevin Rooney, and one of our best Olympic champions, Davey Moore. (Unfortunately, Moore won one championship fight and then died in a freak auto accident in his own driveway.) Arum set up a perfectly awful fight between our heavyweight Olympian, who turned out to be a steroid junkie, and a tall, skinny boxer whose claim to fame was that he had good credentials in track. That alone should have told her something.

Johnson insisted on this dog instead of a fight between Rooney and Moore, another spitfire. Well, I turned it down flat, and Arum, being the snake that he is, took it to the producer behind my back. Apparently he had never really believed that mine was the final word in boxing matters.

The producer reacted just like the rest of the TV executives. All she heard was Arum telling her he had heavyweights on tap for a great fight. Even though we had the Rooney fight in the can—a great six-round fight. It had timed out perfectly. No contest. Besides which, I'd given Arum a flat no.

Imagine my indignation when I found out Albert and I had to call a perfectly awful heavyweight fight, which featured more running than in the Millrose games. It was a huge yawn and a resounding embarrassment.

Not conversant with TV cover-up and etiquette, I went on the air in our wrap-up and blasted away.

"I apologize to our boxing audience. We had a great Rooney–Moore fight to show, that went the full six rounds in an unbelievable toe-to-toe fight, but our producer chose to show you that last stinkeroo."

Cohen's eyes were bulging and his mouth was opened wide when I went off the air.

"Man, you just criticized your own network, your producer. Are you suicidal?"

"I just tell them like it is. What the producer did was major-league dumb."

"What you did was dumber," Cohen grumbled into his hot dog.

As we were lined up to board our plane, Cohen came to me with a worried look on his pudgy face.

"Ohlmeyer is on the phone and boy, is he hot."

I decided to do what I always do when I feel I'm right. I didn't give him a chance to speak. I launched into an attack on the entire program, telling him it was a major mess, and what was worse, it was my face on camera taking the heat.

Ohlmeyer finally got to respond. He had started off with a roar, but now he was quiet and reasonable.

"All I'm saying, Ferdie, is you never point out our mistakes on camera. The producer didn't know she wasn't supposed to listen to Arum, and that you had the last word. All I'm saying is, let's keep our family squabbles in our house. Don't air our dirty laundry."

"Well, in that case, you're right, and I apologize," I said, satisfied.

"Forget it," he said, and hung up. I never heard another word from him, her, or her successor.

✗✗✗✗✗✗

Let me state clearly that had it not been for Barry Frank and his friendship with Don Ohlmeyer, I would never have been in a position to help boxing on TV, to help affect boxing safety measures, and to accomplish all the other things I do in my life even now.

They are both powerful men, but they still have the same faults and frailties as all of us, and when it comes down to it, I owe what I became in TV sports to these two men. Period.

CHAPTER 13

The Fun and Pain of Boxing

By 1981 boxing had done very well in the ratings, and creatively I think we did things never before tried. We had a ball thinking up zany openings and doing anything for a laugh. We enjoyed what we were doing, and it showed in our work. Of course, the best part for me was being able to say whatever I wanted when I sat in front of the mike.

Besides the brilliant Mike Weisman, who was moving up in his career and was soon to be too big to bother with boxing, we had a group of rising young producers who were following in his footsteps.

Peter Rolfe was a model-handsome young man who was excellent because of his solid work ethic and attention to detail. He loved producing boxing shows because of the freedom it gave him to travel.

David Neal, the crown prince of NBC, had the Weisman touch. He always strove to be thoroughly prepared, but if something did go wrong, he was swift in making it right. Neal and I traveled to Africa together for a return to the Rumble in the Jungle, and we filmed the 25th anniversary of the Clay–Liston fight, which won an Emmy. Neal is definitely the future of NBC sports.

Ted Nathanson, scion of a department store family, was a slow, fuddy-duddy, dawdling old man, who was best at pro football. I don't think he ever got used to boxing. He was promoted to executive producer of NBC Sports.

Every show must go through the hands of a director, and here we got very lucky with the multifaceted John Gonzalez. He had been trained in baseball under the legendary Harry Coyle, an ex-B-17 bomber pilot. His touch was so sure that NBC gave him the Super Bowl to direct.

Gonzalez had been a musician and singer when he was a teenager and had an around-the-world tour under his belt. He had quite an active mind, which led him to write a mystery novel that revolved around the Super Bowl game. In Gonzalez I found a kindred spirit, because he was interested in art, loved to talk history, and had a great appetite for life.

In general, our crews were top rate. John Fillipelli was a funny kind of New Yorker who hadn't exorcized his demons from Vietnam. Today he heads up an entire sports network. I loved to talk to him about 'Nam and did a couple of pen and inks about it, which I believe are hanging in his cellar. Today, Fillipelli has left ABC, where he was the executive producer, to go to the newly formed New York Sports Cable owned by George Steinbrenner.

Ohlmeyer, the executive producer and pilot light of NBC Sports, had gotten tired of running a network and retired to Hawaii to count his coupons. He had had credentials. He had headed their number-one blockbuster, *Monday Night Football.* He had Cosell, "Dandy Don" Meredith, and Frank Gifford. Ohlmeyer had glitter and pizzazz; he was young, handsome, and aggressive, and enjoyed a big reputation. From what I saw, he did everything he was hired to do, and NBC got more than its money's worth. I found Ohlmeyer great to work with, a guiding hand that left you plenty of room to succeed or fail. If you succeeded, he left you alone. If you failed, you were toast. That is the way to run a network. Bottom line: Ohlmeyer was a big man, period.

I sure missed him when he left. Anarchy took his place. Each producer was his own boss, and NBC president Arthur Watson was like Big Daddy. His soft, avuncular Irish manner made him a great favorite of the troops. During this free-wheeling period, it was a fantastic pleasure to work at NBC.

Watson did dopey things that somehow made him more loveable. For example, he once confided in me that he knew absolutely nothing about boxing, but he said he made up his executive mind by asking the guy who pumped gas into his car every Monday. Watson never saw one *Cross Road Fight!* "You mean," I gasped, "I owe my job to the Shell Oil pump attendant?" Things don't have to make much sense in television.

During this time, NBC executives began to get nervous about the freedom I enjoyed in lining up fights, sealing the deals, and then "calling 'em the way I saw 'em" come time for the fight. This is when Sean McManus first came into the picture. McManus got stuck trying to control me, which was pretty hard for him to do, because, first, he was very young, with scant life experience, and second, he had zero executive experience and less than zero knowledge of boxing. Once, in an effort to insinuate himself into the process, he timidly asked me if I could put a fight together between Larry Holmes and Alexis Arguello! Holmes was the Heavyweight Champion of the World, a huge 250-pound animal, and Arguello was a featherweight—a gnat! Holmes could step on Arguello and squish him.

I wanted to take McManus by the hand and lead him into Watson's office, like a teacher taking a student to see the principal. I figured Watson would then punish him by making him write, "I don't know anything about boxing!" at least 500 times.

Although I held McManus in some disdain and ridicule at first, I must admit I grew to like him, and in time, as he proved himself under fire time and again, I came to respect him. When Ohlmeyer left, they punted McManus over to Frank, who had sold NBC an awful lot of product. Eyebrows were raised again.

Then, during one Orange Bowl, Watson called saying he wanted to come by my house. I was painting a piece for an upcoming art show and told him to come on over.

He sat for an uncomfortable 15 minutes while I painted serenely, my Artie Shaw CD playing full blast. Finally he asked if I'd mind stopping and turning down the music, which I did, and he launched into what seemed a very uncomfortable subject for him. He said the "Big Boys" wanted some financial control over me, and they'd like to get an executive with accounting experience to monitor my deals.

I said matter-of-factly that I'd do them one better than that. I'd quit and they could make the deals; I'd just call the fights.

At the time, there was a violent cry from the New York press that what I was doing showed a blatant conflict of interest. By organizing fights that I would then critique on camera smelled to high heaven, and God knows, I agreed with them. My comment was that the writers should scrutinize each and every fight, and if they ever caught me in an improper commentary they should blast me, and I'd agree with them in print. None of them ever did, but let's face it, it was wrong. However, I've always been very honest and straightforward. If a fight is bad, I say it stinks! If it's good, it's good, no matter who set up the fight.

When he got back to New York, Watson put McManus and his keeper, Bert Zeldin the accountant, on a plane to come to Miami and meet with me and read me the riot act. I gleefully awaited their arrival.

I went to pick them up and took the long way home through Coral Gables, down Coconut Drive, through downtown and finally to my home in Bay Point. That ate up some time and gave them a regal ride as well.

My beautiful wife, Luisita, had decked out our house with fresh flowers, the paintings on the wall were lit for display, and the house smelled of delicious culinary aromas. It was truly a showplace.

We had lunch, and I regaled them with stories, none of which had to do with boxing or NBC. The meal was superb, and then we barely had time to get back to the airport. They were filled with good food, good wine, and good cheer. I drove them straight to Miami International, suggested they order a subscription to *Ring* magazine, and then put them on the plane. They hadn't gotten a word in edgewise.

The next day Watson called. I couldn't tell if he was sputtering mad or laughing at himself. "You bastard! I should have known better than to send them to talk to you."

I laughed and told him, "You should get a subscription to *Ring* magazine, too, just keep talking to the guy who pumps your gas and call me back when you grow up."

He was laughing when I hung up. What a guy.

The next shot Watson took at me was so bad it was comical. I had arranged a superb fight in England between Marvin Hagler and a tough Englishman by the name of Alan Minter. It figured to become a real brawl. The fight was held in Manchester, where working class blokes take their boxing seriously and throw bottles when their man loses, so it wasn't a place for the faint of heart.

We had just finished our opening spot and sat down in our spiffy new tuxes when I felt somebody sit down next to me. I was shocked to see it was McManus. He looked at me with what I could best discern as his most serious, no-nonsense face.

"What the hell are you doing here?" I asked him.

"This fight better be good or else," he said, manfully lowering his voice an octave and ignoring my question. It was all I could do to keep from laughing.

It was seconds to airtime and here was this amateur throwing meaningless ultimatums at me.

"Or else what, Sean? You gonna take my passport and strand me in England for life?"

He blinked a few times, not knowing what to say to back up this statement.

"Don't ever talk to me again when we're doing a show. This may be the fight of the year, but if it's not, tough shit!" I said, shooing him out of the booth.

Hagler knocked out Minter in three brawling rounds, and I don't think I ever saw McManus in Europe again, or anywhere else for that matter.

I'll never understand why Watson threw this wet-behind-the-ears kid at me; I just couldn't see the sense in it. And I felt sorry for McManus. How could a kid control an old warhorse like me?

Rahway Penitentiary, "The Animal," and Others

Murray Gaby, Lou Esa's manager, had very solid political connections in the New Jersey Penal System through his brother, who was very close to the governor. There was a ticking time bomb in Rahway Penitentiary by the name of James Scotty Scott, a.k.a. "Great Scott." He had been part of the prison population since he was 12 and was a pure prison jungle cat. Scott was a light heavyweight, and man could he fight. There were few better than he.

I found out about him through Gaby, and we hatched a plot to televise boxing out of the pen. The warden was always looking for good publicity, so he liked the idea. At the time, Watson's gas-pumping adviser must have been on vacation, and even their lawyers must have been asleep, because I snuck this proposal in, and amazingly we had our A-Team with Weisman-Gonzalez and our All-Stars at the prison.

The setting was grim, but Scott was the king of the joint, so we were well protected in an odd sort of way. I even felt safe enough to bring my wife, along with Weisman's sister-in-law, both drop-dead gorgeous, and none of the prisoners so much as looked at them.

We aired six fights; all victories for Scott, and although he was a hardened criminal with a rap sheet as long as the *Gone With the Wind* manuscript, the state of New Jersey saw fit to parole him into Gaby's care in Miami.

Well, a man who has spent his entire adult life behind bars does not find his way around freedom easily. After two days in Miami, I took Scott out to eat at Wolfie's on South Beach and found he hadn't eaten the entire time. When I asked him why, he told me that nobody had told him to. I felt like a fool, especially after I watched as he finished off a big turkey dinner, wiped his utensils clean with his napkin, and then stood up and put the spoon in his back pocket.

"No, no, Scotty. We leave the utensils here," I said, fighting my urge to crack a joke.

I knew better than that. I also found out that he needed to be told when to go to sleep and wake up. His toilet habits, well, he handled those on his own. Whew!

At the time I had a nice friendship going with Jimmy Johnson, the mercurial head coach of the undefeated Miami Hurricanes. We were mutual admirers, so I felt it would be nice if Scott saw a college football game at the Orange Bowl. Johnson was kind enough to suggest we watch from the sidelines. Scott was excited as he walked among the huge Miami ballplayers and gawked at the leggy cheerleaders. He even appreciated the loud band music and the screaming crowd. I settled him down in the corner of the end zone as Miami was marching down the field to score, and score they did. Everyone whooped and hollered, and then the team's cannon, Touchdown Tommy, went off with a deafening ka-boom! Scott ducked, and then turned and fled for the exit. It took me an hour to find him—he was hiding under the stands—and explain to him that no one was shooting at him; he was perfectly safe. Well, he never asked me to take him to another game.

✗✗✗✗✗✗

Gaby, pulling every string in the book, got Scott a championship fight in England! Against all odds, he had managed to get Scott six fights in jail, get him paroled, and now, a title fight. What a great accomplishment. But, alas, it was not to be! Generous, well-intentioned Gaby made a big mistake before it ever materialized. He bought Scott an old Pontiac, and the ex-con's new set of wheels became bad news. In less time than it takes me to write this, Scott jumped in his car and made a break for his old New Jersey stomping grounds to follow some strange religious sect he was involved with in prison. They were radical and violent, and according to him, the leaders had instructed him to kill an old enemy of the sect. Scott shot the man dead. Of course, he claimed to have loaned the Pontiac to his cousin, swearing they looked identical, except that his cousin didn't have his mean left hook. Unfortunately, a witness saw the crime unfold from across the street, and it didn't help that the witness was a guard at Rahway Penitentiary, who knew Scott well. Scott said the white guard was mistaken; all blacks look the same to white folks. The problem there was that the guard was black, too.

Kachunk! The prison bars clanked shut behind the "Great Scott," and not even Gaby, a title shot, or the power of NBC could get him out. James Scott is still in Rahway and will be there for a long time after this story is told.

✗✗✗✗✗✗

We booked Frank "The Animal" Fletcher on our shows broadcast from Atlantic City. He was an immediate hit, because he really was an animal; at least he fought like one. And he brought a side attraction with him, his mother. She'd show up at ringside, hugging a giant Panda bear wrapped in cellophane to keep her son's blood splatterings from ruining it.

As the public caught on to Fletcher, their interest in his mother piqued and we started receiving mail about her. She was a riot, running around the ring, yelling and screaming, and clutching the plastic-covered panda. All of our fans wanted us to interview her, but Fletcher would have none of it. He kept winning, she kept dragging around that bear, and the public kept asking to know more.

One day I caught Fletcher coming in from his roadwork and pinned him down. "'Animal,' why don't you let us do a piece on your mother?"

"Aw, man," he said, hanging his head, "she ain't my mother. I just rent her."

I thought I had heard it all, but that was a new one, and it closed the case for me. As Chris Dundee always said, "There ain't no George Washingtons in boxing."

✗✗✗✗✗✗

I did an awful lot of business with the Duva family. First of all, they were a legitimate boxing family. Lou and his brother had been tough guys for the Teamsters under Jimmy Hoffa. They boxed, and then they trained, managed, and finally promoted boxing around Totowa, New Jersey.

Lou Duva was an old pal. He was short and round. In those days, Harry James had a hit record called "Mister Five By Five." That was Lou. His face looked like an English bulldog. Chris Dundee had introduced me and told me to depend on Lou. I did, and NBC got many a great show from him.

By the time I started using Duva's fighters, he had brought along his son Dan to promote. Dan Duva was a bright lawyer who only resembled his father physically. He was calm, quiet, and cerebral; a great counterbalance to Lou's mercurial personality. Dan's wife, Kathy, was brainy, so they put her in charge of the press, and she was great. Lou had other children and put all of them to work in his company. It was a solid family enterprise and a great team of professionals to work with.

The Duvas had a ball of muscle fighter named Frankie Warren, and I was high on him if for no other reason than what he did for me by shutting up that mountainous mass of misinformation, Mike Katz of *The New York Times*.

Katz was a short, heavyset man with a huge beard and wild bushy hair that came to his shoulders. Like most of New York, he had fallen in love with a slick fighter named Buddy McGirt and was already assigning him ring immortality, naming him pound for pound as the best and all of those silly titles, which rightfully belong in a sports bar. To hardcore boxing people, a pound-for-pound compliment is accorded to great fighters at the end of a successful career, not in mid-career. Legitimate pound for pounds are Sugar Ray Robinson, Willie Pep, Roberto Duran, etc.

Katz accosted me in the Garden one time while I was watching a fight with NBC media relations guru Kevin Monaghan.

"Why are you ducking Buddy McGirt?" Katz snarled at me. "Why won't you put him in with Frankie Warren?"

I was taken aback, because I was not a boxing promoter, but only a boxing consultant. I didn't make fights. I had no favorite fighters to protect. I just looked at the fat, unkempt Katz and said, "Across the ring from us is Danny Duva. He manages Warren, and he's the promoter for Main Events. Walk over and tell him I'll give him an NBC-TV date if you make the match."

Katz waddled around the ring and accosted Duva, who immediately accepted the match, no problem. Buddy McGirt versus Frankie Warren was a peach of a fight because McGirt was an excellent fighter, but I didn't think he had enough experience to hang in with a tough kid like Frankie Warren. The fact that McGirt was undefeated and touted by all of the New York writers as a pound-for-pound blah would make for a big rating. I laughed at Katz. If he wanted to get his darling beat to satisfy his ego, okay, I'd oblige him.

On July 20, 1986, Warren beat McGirt soundly, and I didn't hear a peep from the corpulent Katz until one night, months later, when he had suffered one of his periodic attacks of amnesia after he had been wrong, once again, in *The New York Times*.

"You guys at NBC think you got such a hot shot in Alex Ramos. Well, I got a guy in California, J.C. Williamson, who'll knock out Ramos."

"What? Again?" I looked at him in disgust. "Why don't you leave making fights to real boxing people and confine yourself to your writing?"

He persisted, getting hot and bothered and riled up. So, once again I said, "Okay, it's an easy win for Ramos."

Net result: Ramos won an easy 10-round decision, and Katz retired from matchmaking.

✗✗✗✗✗✗

New York boxing writers are a rare breed. It's hard to conceive how a body of men can be so filled with their own importance, in spite of the number of times they are wrong. They are called experts, which does not carry with it the burden of being right most of the time, but apparently only means you have a job writing about boxing. Watson's gas-pumper would be a boxing expert, if someone would give him a typewriter and a job.

Being a writer for a long time, I idolized a lot of writers, even if they were from New York City. My best friend and a man who is still my idol is Budd Schulberg. He really knows boxing. Red Smith of *The New York Times,* when he came slumming into our ranks, was the Dean. Old timers loved boxing. Most of them were on the take, although it's not fashionable to admit it now. I came in on the tail end of it. When we'd bring a boxer to fight in the Garden, Angelo held court in his room, handing $50 bills to every boxing writer in New York. There were more than three newspapers at the time.

Fifty from the opposing fighter matched the $50 we handed out. So what did we get out of it? This bought the sportswriter's guarantee that he would write a "fair" story about the fight. Is it any wonder that I treated the New York sports press with somewhat less respect than they thought I should show them?

I knew all of the press and treated them kindly during the Ali years—people of high reputations, like Red Smith, Dave Anderson, Wilfred Sheed, and Ring Lardner Jr. I was in awe of and helped them wherever I could, giving them access to Ali when no one else could get to him.

When NBC hired me, the reception turned decidedly frosty from the New York press. I became the enemy. One of the writers I had befriended was Barney Nagler, a very short, professional type, who smoked pipes, wore button-down shirts and black ties with sleeveless sweaters. I think he was trying to look like an Ivy League professor. He'd suffered a bout with cancer of the lower colon, and had been operated on, so anytime he saw me, he gave me a full report on his medical condition, including the color of his stool and much more detailed information than I needed to know. I was always courteous and listened attentively, and gave him encouraging pep talks.

One day at a press conference, I greeted him cordially, waiting to get his medical report, and he verbally attacked me.

"Who do you think you are? How dare you apply for the job of boxing consultant at NBC? Why, in the days of the IBC, I was the boxing consultant. I should have been hired. What qualifications do you bring to the job?"

I stood open-mouthed, being raked over the coals by this little man for nothing I was aware of, except being hired for a job he thought he had the right to. From then until he died, he barely spoke to me, and he wrote and spoke of me in the most derogatory of terms. Because he was so short, I had no trouble overlooking him.

Nagler decided to write a tell-all book about the International Boxing Club, which ran boxing like a monopoly. Nagler was the paid go-between for NBC. What he did with this book was rat out his former bosses, a lawyer named Truman Gibson, and a Chicago millionaire, James Norris, who was a boxing aficionado and didn't need the illegal strategies they used, which eventually landed all of them in the penitentiary.

When I brought the book to Chris Dundee, he almost went through the ceiling. Chris was still steaming over the story Nagler told over and over about the time Nagler was trying to find Carbo to do a story and was having a hard time finding him. Chris was a manager/fighter/promoter with connections. He lived in the Lexington Hotel, across from the automat where Carbo had breakfast every morning.

"Do you know Frankie Carbo?" Nagler asked.

"No," said Chris, not looking up from the *Ring* magazine he was reading.

"He eats across the street where you have breakfast."

"So?"

"You don't know him?" Nagler asked incredulously. "You're in boxing, and you don't know about him?"

"I know he has two doughnuts every morning," said Chris, trying to act helpful. Not many people in the hard days of the 1930s had money for two sinkers.

"So you can't tell me where to find him?"

"Call the lost and found," said Chris, motioning Nagler to go away, as one would a pesky fly.

Discouraged, Nagler walked out of the small, dingy room, but when he got to the door, he felt the urge to urinate. He opened the bathroom door and almost fainted. There stood Carbo in his undershirt, shaving! Chris hated that story.

"Why that little prick! He was the first in line of New York writers taking payoffs. We paid him $150 a week." Chris's glasses were steaming over. "And he didn't miss one week!"

It was October 1970, and we were going to the Jerry Quarry–Ali fight in Atlanta. Chris got off the plane and steamed right into the press room, where he made a beeline for the card game where Nagler was playing. Chris was already an old man, but it was all I could do to physically restrain him from giving Nagler a sound beating. He accused Nagler of lying, cheating, and being a play-for-pay ratfink.

Nagler didn't answer, cowering behind some bigger writers. He sunk beneath contemptible in my book. I don't mind a crook. I mind a rat.

This brings us back to the hard-to-understand behavior of *New York Times* writer Mike Katz. Once I saved Katz from going to a Las Vegas jail and missing a deadline. He had barged into the press room to file his story, and a Las Vegas sheriff had detained him because he had no press pass.

Katz got on his New York high horse, blustering a tirade at the officer, who calmly handcuffed him and was leading him to jail. I intervened and in a calm way tried to reason with the policeman and tell him Katz had a job to do, and he would get fired if he missed the deadline. I ran out and got Arum, who is a lawyer as well as a promoter for the fight. It took all we could do to get Katz to his typewriter.

I don't know about Arum, but I never got even a thank-you nod. Not that I expected any, for most New York reporters who are imbued with a rude attitude that precludes issuing a simple thank you. Katz turned in the example of any rude, disgraceful, and unthankful piece of behavior any writer in my 40 years of sports. He was in Miami with his wife and was faced with a genuine life-or-death catastrophe. He called my home and sounded in acute distress. His wife had advanced breast cancer and had spent the night in agonizing pain as she hemorrhaged. It was a Sunday in a strange town, and he was facing a very expensive medical emergency.

I immediately called a great friend, Dr. Howard Gordon, who is a world-famous plastic surgeon. His office had its own private surgical suite. I asked for his help, and as he always did for me, he left his family and came to his office. He had to call his nurse to assist us, and I went to the Fontainebleau Hotel to pick up the suffering Mrs. Katz.

The work took the better part of an hour. She was in poor shape. If she could stand a plane trip, she should return to New York City and be admitted to a New York hospital. In order to save ambulance, fees, etc., I stayed with them and drove her to Miami International Airport. I filled her full of painkillers and got her on the plane, and then wished them good luck.

The disease was far advanced, and unfortunately she didn't last very long. I never heard a word of thanks or a note of appreciation from Katz. If Gordon and I had charged our normal fees, plus nursing fees, plus operating room costs and transportation, it would have cost between $5,000 and $10,000, easy.

Although I didn't expect an offer to defray costs, I think a nice letter to Dr. Gordon was in order, and further, I thought I had extracted a thorn from the lion's paw and would not suffer further slings and arrows from Katz's shabby typewriter.

How wrong I was. One day all of New York called me to say Katz had written that I had lost my medical license to practice. This was directly traceable to Arum, whose evil tongue knows no bound. To make it more ludicrous, I had just received the highest award for my medical work in the ghetto from the Governor of Florida, Bob Martinez!

I am not by nature (or disposition) a litigious person, but I must admit, in the light of our life-saving medical favor, it was a bit much. I settled for a retraction in the paper, because I thought so little of lawyers and lawsuits, and because I thought even less of Mike Katz.

The Letterman Debacle

One Cohen masterpiece backfired splendidly, and what a crash it was! For a few years I had been trying to get NBC exposure on night television for our big shows, all to no avail. Not even Cohen could get us space.

Late-night host David Letterman was starting to catch on, but the most he would do was put on Marv Albert, who had a series of TV sports goofs he played. But Albert was not born to the streets of hustle, and he felt he was lowering himself to plug NBC's upcoming fights. Albert was a great self-promoter but was weak when it came to mentioning others.

On the other hand, Letterman delighted in having on Don King, the sworn enemy of NBC boxing. At the time, King was so pissed at me that he threatened a $15 million lawsuit against NBC. I couldn't get on to promote a major primetime fight, but King could get on to trash us. It was unbelievable self-flagellation on the part of NBC.

We had finally stolen Holmes, the heavyweight champ, from King and his WBC partners. We had him in a great primetime fight. It was a kind of test-the-water fight to see if primetime would pay for itself. NBC needed to get on Letterman and plug it.

I arrived backstage at the David Letterman show at 3 p.m., ahead of schedule, to make sure all was set. The first guy to greet me was the producer.

"What funny stories are you going to tell? You're going to tell some Ali stories, I'm sure. And, oh, by the way, you're not going to mention Don King."

"I was under the impression that Dave would ask me what he wants, and then I'd get into our primetime promo," I said cautiously. The producer nodded distractedly and scuttled off down the hall.

An hour later, as I was going through makeup, a quiet, mousy man with a rubber briefcase showed up. I've always been wary of guys carrying rubber briefcases. (It's an Ybor City thing.)

"We're almost ready," he began, and I nodded. "Oh, by the way, you're not going to mention Don King, are you?" he asked worriedly.

"Not unless Dave brings it up," I smiled a bleak smile.

He turned out to be the censor for NBC.

I progressed to the Green Room, hob-knobbing with the hoi polloi, when two three-button suit guys came in with leather briefcases.

"We're here from the legal department," began the tall man cheerfully, "and we just want to be sure you are not going to mention Don King."

By this time, I was on fire. Now all I wanted to talk about was Don King.

The time came and I found myself standing offstage in the wings, next to David Letterman. Now, for years I'd seen him in the halls. He'd always been cordial, and I the same. I can't say we were friends, but he knew who I was, and I knew who he was. We eyed one another. I gave a cheerful "Hi, Dave" sort of wave. He eyed me coldly and said nothing at all. It was as if I had come to serve him a subpoena. His iceberg demeanor stunned me.

Up music! Up lights! Letterman bounces into an ear-splitting oration and begins, "Tonight I have the great pleasure to introduce you to the voice of boxing on radio and TV. For years it was the highlight of my life to sit on my father's knee and listen to this man describe fights on Friday night. Please welcome 'The Fight Doctor,' Ferdie Pacheco."

There was polite applause. I was steaming. Fuck this pompous prick, I thought, as I took my chair by his desk. Letterman did a trick with his pencil and smiled warmly at me.

"First of all, David, if I was the highlight of your life, you must have had a dreary life. Secondly, I was never on radio. You were listening to Don Dunphy."

Letterman looked confused, like he had no reason why I was attacking him.

"You sound mad. What are you mad about?" he said defensively.

I described the three-time threats about King by his minions, and he graciously told me, "Mention Don King all you like. Hell, we'll assume the legal bills."

The interview was a shambles, because all we did talk about was King. We broke for a two-minute commercial and immediately Letterman turned on the ice machine again. I got down to business.

"I'm here to sell Monday's show on primetime with Larry Holmes. When do we get to that?"

"Don't worry. We have two minutes when we get back. We'll hop right into it."

Music! Lights! We're back, ice melts, Letterman looks at me as if he loves me.

"Doc, you've been in boxing for over 30 years, you actually worked corners, trained fighters, and were, in fact, a fight doctor. So, here is a question I have been dying to ask you for years. It's about boxers fooling around before a fight."

He did a trick with his pencil.

"Fooling around? What does that mean?" I feigned innocence and Letterman looked stricken.

"You know, with a girl."

"A girl?" Again I gave a blank stare.

"You know, um, is a boxer celibate before a fight?"

"What is celibate? Is that an Italian wine?"

The audience was on to what I was doing, and Letterman started to catch on. He wasn't happy. People were laughing, but *at* him. He dropped his pencil.

"I mean does he get laid before a fight?"

"No," I said and didn't expand on the topic.

I had had two minutes to get my promo in and now all of the time was gone. I got up to leave cold David Letterman trying to figure out what went wrong.

"Great interview," said Cohen sarcastically. "I especially liked the part about the Larry Holmes fight this Monday."

But in the end, he laughed. I never ever made it back to *The David Letterman Show,* but King did. Albert and his goof reel did. I didn't. I wonder why.

CHAPTER 14

NBC Gags and Screenwriting

We were on a roll with our *Sportsworld* shows on NBC and were being left on our own by the executives. I was booking great fights at bargain basement prices, the ratings were high, and as far as production value, the returns were the best in the business due to Weisman and his amazing production team. The creative energy of our team took a turn toward comedy that became a staple for our show.

The gags started innocently enough when we hatched an opening we called "Absent Marv." This became a running gag that Albert wouldn't even have to participate in, which suited him just fine. One time we were in Paris for a fight and we dug up a smelly street drunk, sat him in a chair next to me at a sidewalk café in Montmarte, and gave him an absinthe to drink. I talked to him just like I would to Albert.

The scene opened with the cameras rolling on a closeup of me.

"We've been in Paris three riotous days and nights, and we've partied hard, but now it's back to work. As usual, I'm with my broadcast partner, Marv Albert."

The camera panned out to show the drunk, slobbering over his absinthe, and then back to me

"Do you think Marcel 'the boxer' has a chance over Burton 'the puncher?'"

Again the cameras closed in on him. The old derelict snarled at the lens and then let out a long, loud belch. Talk about a potent editorial comment!

Once, in Tampa, I was seated at the end of a long pier with the camera closeup on me.

"Isn't this a wonderful view of Tampa Bay, Marv?" I said, and I swept my arm exaggeratedly out over the vista just as one of the assistants dropped a huge piece of concrete into the bay. Just by chance, the water splashed up where Albert was supposed to be, and the camera caught it perfectly.

"Marv? Marv?" I said, acting really startled, getting louder and louder. "Oh no! Marv!" I craned down over the railing. "Man overboard!" I yelled.

The longer we did these stunts, the wilder they got. I can't say Albert was pleased, because his image was being used for something akin to stupid pet tricks, but he was never there anyway. Besides, the general consensus was that Albert always took himself too seriously. He didn't want to appear any more foolish than a man with an ill-fitting toupee could.

One gag we never got to do, and I regret it to this day, was for me to be made up like a ventriloquist's dummy and sit on Albert's lap. His deep, distinguished voice would come out of my flapping jaws to say, "Today! Live at Caesar's Palace in Las Vegas! It's *Sportsworld!*"

Well, Albert finally put his foot down and refused to do it. Too bad, it could have been a classic.

Another favorite of mine, which unfortunately didn't make it into the show, took place in the middle of a Tampa bakery. Somehow, the idea of starting a *Sportsworld* show in a bakery appealed to my sense of the absurd, not to mention my sweet tooth. Phil Alessi, a bakery owner and local fight promoter, was more than willing to pull off this stunt with me.

We opened the show with a big introduction of Alessi as he beamed his appreciation. He offered up a tray of huge strawberry cream puffs and put them down between us. The camera shot a closeup of Alessi as he answered my first question. Then it panned back to me. My mouth was covered with whipped cream and strawberries, but I acted as if nothing was wrong, and asked the next question, followed by another closeup of Alessi, answering with a completely straight face.

When the camera came back to me, strawberries and cream were now up to my eyeglasses, but I went on as usual and asked Alessi the next question. He never cracked a smile. What a deadpan. Get it? Bakery? Deadpan?

The final shot was the best. My entire face, up to my hairline, was covered with the confection, and the only thing you could see was my mouth moving.

"Thanks, Phil Alessi. And now, from Tampa, Florida, it's *Sportsworld!*"

Unfortunately, my comic cohort wasn't there to rescue me that day, and the scene was axed for fear of executive reprisal, using the lame excuse that it looked like I was shaving and had cut myself. How do these people make a living?

Perhaps our most shameful stunt was pulled when there was a big brouhaha brewing over a low blow that had stopped a big fight. Looking into my history books I found that Foul-Proof Taylor who had invented the protective boxer's cup tested the prototype by going around the streets of New York with a baseball bat, asking people to hit him in the crotch with it! He did this until the boxing commission gave in and adopted the cup, which is worn to this day to ward off the possibility of a fight being stopped because of a low blow.

In spite of the invention, we had just such an incident happen in the previous week's fight, so I convinced Weisman to outfit one of our assistants with a cup and have a boxer slam him with a bat. Naturally, Weisman liked the idea, but when we turned to the sullen crew and asked for volunteers all we got were adamant rejections. So Weisman, who took no mercy on women in sportscasting, turned to a female crew member by the name of Mary Ann, who stood there convinced she was exempt from his craziness.

"Mary Ann will do it." Then, smiling his best Kermit the Frog smile at her, he said, "She's got nothing to lose."

Mary Ann was a favorite with the crew. She was bright as hell and always went out of her way to help on a show. She would have won any popularity contest, but as far as looks, she wasn't pretty; she was just one of the guys. However, the girl did have a great set of legs—a $9^1/_2$ on a scale of 10, to be sure, but they were offset by the frazzled, cut-off jeans and big combat boots she wore like her male counterparts. And she never used makeup or combed her hair unless it was absolutely necessary.

Luckily for us, Mary Ann was a good sport, too. So we busily arranged for her to step into the big red leather crotch protector. Unfortunately, our boxer, the designated hitter, refused to swing at her, as did everybody else. It was beginning to look like she'd have to take a swing at herself—a kind of pelvic suicide, which you could tell she wasn't exactly thrilled with. Then, a volunteer emerged. He took a swing, but it was just a tap.

"No good," Weisman said. "You're pulling the swing. Hit it like you're hitting a home run!"

Whap! Mary Ann stood there blinking as I huddled with Weisman, watching.

"You know what? The fact that she's a girl kinda takes the wind out of the sails," I said, as Weisman's eyes opened wide, a signal that he'd come up with one of his brilliant ideas.

"How about if you introduce the piece by telling that crazy history of the cup, then when the guy swings, there'll be a fresh egg in it."

"That would work!" I happily agreed.

Mary Ann was dressed in her usual tattered and extremely short cutoffs, with her combat boots and big roll-down socks. The camera-man focused in on her legs and gave a long whistle as Weisman and I looked at them through the viewfinder. They looked great on camera. Then, with his best Kermit smile, he signaled for the batter to swing.

Whap! The runny egg white started to ooze down her gorgeous gams, followed by the sticky yellow yolk. The crew gasped as tears welled up in Mary Ann's eyes and onlookers gave out a chorus of "Oooeee, gooey! Yuk!"

Weisman was nonplussed.

"We need a hard-boiled egg!" he called out.

Mary Ann, looking up from toweling off the sticky mess, was silently seething.

"You know, Mike," I offered. "The only thing we're proving here is that the belt doesn't protect you."

"That'll be our fallback position," he said.

You could tell he was driven to succeed, no matter what turn a story took.

Then, with the boiled egg nestled in the big cup between Mary Ann's lovely legs, the batter swung. Whap! Pieces of crumbled egg and shell started falling to the floor. Disconsolate, we stared at each other. Then my friend Phil Alessi came up with a white marble egg he used as a paperweight.

"Eureka!" we both said. Even Mary Ann was laughing in relief, glad that the end of her agony was in sight.

Solemnly, I went on camera holding the "chicken" egg, telling all of America how safe the protective cup is and that we would demonstrate by striking it full force with a Louisville Slugger. The egg was then put in Mary Ann's cup, the batter wound up and whap! Nothing happened, luckily, and the egg was taken out, unbroken. So much for truth in broadcasting!

Poor Mary Ann, her face was never seen on camera, but her gorgeous gams were plastered all over national TV. I wonder how many fans even discerned that the cup was attached to a girl. I figured you'd have to be blind not to connect those perfect legs with a female, but, as H.L. Mencken once said, "You'll never go wrong underestimating the intelligence of the average sports fan."

✗✗✗✗✗✗✗

When our shows were set in Las Vegas, I would prevail on stand-up comics to open for us. Instead of a big NBC opening, we'd have Jackie Mason sitting in an easy chair, talking to the audience and saying something like, "Hey, you! Whaddaya doin' sittin' on the sofa watching this nonsense? Haven't you got anything better to do than watch a Mexican and a Jew fight? Ain't the sun shining where you're at? Get up, turn off the set, go outside, and play with your kid. All you're gonna get here is a New York Jew with a bad rug, who don't know a thing about boxing, fightin' with some 'Spic doctor, who don't know any more than the Jew. Go, take my word for it, you ain't missin' a thing."

Then, from the announcer would come, "Live from the MGM Grand in Las Vegas, its *Sportsworld!*" Followed by a swell of opening music.

Weisman loved it. Once, we even had the deadpan one-linemeister Henny Youngman with his violin, telling his 30-year-old boxing jokes to a rapt audience. He was most definitely a brilliant comic.

When we were really on a roll with our openings, we had to face a mini-crisis. I wanted Shecky Green for the segment, but it was a last-minute call and he wasn't available. Looking in the newspaper, I read that Susan Anton was appearing at the Sands Hotel, and on the bill with her was my old friend and former patient, comedian Alan King.

I asked Weisman, "How about this? We do a little camera trick with Susan Anton. Marv will be on one side of her and I'll be on the other, but we'll be so small, we won't even come up to her knees. She'll look like a gorgeous giant! The camera will pan slowly up her legs, all the way up her front to her face and those 150 gleaming front teeth. Then she'll announce, 'From the beautiful Sands Hotel in Las Vegas on the strip, we present ... LIVE ... *SPORTSWORLD!*' What do you think?"

Weisman got up and paced the room. I could tell he liked the idea, but he knew it could generate some feminist criticism. "She *is* tall," he thought out loud.

"And Marv *is* short," I said, chuckling to myself.

After a long pause, he said, "Fuck the feminists. We'll make sure not to linger on the crotch, and besides, she needs the publicity. Do it! Go to the Sands and bag Susan."

I arrived at the Sands between shows and was rudely rebuffed by her manager and a security guard. Anton could not see me, I was told. She was resting between shows to preserve her talent.

"Talent?" I asked naïvely. Her manager gave me the fisheye.

I was pissed. Anton had just started in Vegas, and she could use a good spot on national TV in front of 20 million viewers. Oh, all right, 10 million.

"Well, tell her NBC was here with an offer, but since her rest is more important than her career, tell her to go fu—"

"What's the matter, Doc?" King walked up before I could complete my thought. "Trouble with the broad?" His eyes rolled up to a billboard with Anton's picture plastered all over it.

"I just got turned down by Susan Anton. Susan Anton, for Chrissakes! My life is going downhill fast," I said morosely.

"She's just a kid. She doesn't know yet," he put his arm around me. "Let's go to the bar and have a drink."

We hadn't had the first drink when King turned to me and said, "I hear you're a writer now."

"You mean books?" I said, amazed that King would even know this.

"No, film scripts. I'm looking for a fresh script. I got a three-picture deal cooking and I'm just wrapping up my new movie, *Wolffen,* so I need a third script to start developing. You got anything?"

"Of course," I said with false confidence, my mind racing to come up with a feasible story line. This serendipitous turn of events—and my ability to bullshit—is how I got into screenwriting in the first place.

"Okay, we got time. I'm listening."

I gulped my drink.

"Well, it's a war story, a black comedy," I said, wondering where I was going with it. If I could vamp it out now, I knew I could think up the plot later.

"Kind of like *M.A.S.H.* and *One Flew Over the Cuckoo's Nest* rolled into one."

"Wow! That's great. Give me more." He was on the edge of his seat, and little did he know, so was I.

Now, I had the highest respect for King. His comedic talents were phenomenal, and as a monologist, there were none better. But I was having trouble thinking of him as a film producer. How could I take him seriously? On the other hand, he must have been looking at me thinking, "This guy was my doctor. He's seen me naked!" Now, I ask you, how could he take me seriously, either? But, half of pulling something off on a moment's notice is looking like you know what you're doing, and I must admit, I've always been good at that, so I continued.

"The time is World War II. It has just started and already Rommel has slaughtered the green American troops at Kasserene Pass. Casualties are huge. The Army is not prepared for so many, so they call out any kind of doctors they can get to rush to the field hospitals and do what they can.

"Next we see two doctors in a Jeep on a dusty desert road, headed for the field hospital. One is Dr. Jules Steiner, a Jewish psychiatrist from New York. The other is Frank Garcia, a family doctor from Florida, fresh out of his internship, and he is worried sick.

"'They got me down as a surgeon,' he says. 'I'm not a surgeon, I'm a G.P. I don't have any training in this blood and guts stuff. Christ, I'll kill more guys than I can help!'

"'There, there,' the psychiatrist says in his professional, but condescending manner. 'You'll be better at it than the Arabs they have doing it now.'"

"Arabs?" King says, but I keep on like I haven't heard him.

"At that precise moment, an .88 shell explodes right in front of the Jeep. The doctors leap out, Dr. Steiner to the left, Dr. Garcia to the right. The next shell lands square on Dr. Steiner, and he just vanishes without a trace, not even a belt buckle.

"Then, everything gets quiet, and Frank sits in the Jeep pondering the situation. The psychiatrist is gone, but his briefcase is still on the backseat. Suddenly it dawns on Frank that he may be able to get out of doing surgeries after all. He'll report in as Dr. Steiner and hand them his orders, and then inform them of the untimely death of Dr. Garcia.

"When he reports for duty he finds his patients are mostly combat-fatigued and shell-shocked, but others are obvious malingerers and cowards. It is his job to set up a front-line unit—"

King interrupted. "Like *M.A.S.H.*, only treating nut jobs instead of casualties." He couldn't hide his enthusiasm, but being a New Yorker, he had a healthy skepticism to go along with it.

"You got any of this written down? I'll have to show my production partner."

"Of course," I said, bluffing blindly. I detected that he was bitten and ready to buy. King had one of the sharpest comedic minds in the business, and he had already taken my germ of an idea and started to write it in his head, so I told him, "By the way, Alan. I'll do the writing. I'll give you a synopsis this week and fax it to your New York office. We'll meet there."

It's curious that King was so sold he didn't ask me what the plot was. It was a good thing, though, because I didn't know. It seemed immaterial at the time, like buying a Rolls-Royce by looking at the grill. Oh well, if you're searching for a shallower place than TV sports, you'll find it in the Hollywood, La La Land of movies. They invented shallow.

We shook hands, and I made a note to send Susan Anton a dozen long-stem roses. After all, I owed her for this opportunity.

As soon as I hit my room I called my writing partner, Mimi Roth, in Studio City, California. Mimi was a wonderful, brainy professor of screenwriting at UCLA, who has been in the movie business since her husband, Leon, came out west to be a producer for the Mirisch Company. He made a great movie, *The Luck of Ginger Coffee,* with a wonderful young Irish actor named Richard Harris. Thereafter Leon repaired to Nate and Al's Deli to spin Hollywood yarns about how hard it is to make movies, his credo being, "Making a movie is a battle, getting a movie made is a war."

Leon eventually took a job at USC, teaching screenwriting, and the couple devoted their time to teaching their son, Eric Roth, to be a top-notch screenwriter. Eric became a major talent, writing *Forrest Gump, Airport,* and other mega hits, and is now able to demand million-dollar fees. But that was yet to come. At the time, he was in Little League screenwriters' camp.

Mimi and I had teamed up to write a book based on a prize-winning short story I had written and even used as a Christmas card one year. It was called "Sweet Sam." We had struck a close friendship, and she proceeded to teach me all I know about screenwriting. She was awesome in her knowledge of structure, characters, and plot. And she was a patient, thorough teacher. I could hear her wheels spinning as I told my new story, such as it was, over the phone to her.

"First off," she said, "forget World War II, that's dead at the box office. Next, we set the story in Vietnam. I'll do some research on methods of treatment for shell shock. I'm sure we'll find something. And Julius Steiner, that's his name, is a surgeon, but he hates to operate. Every time he makes an incision, he throws up. That's graphic, and a good opening gag. So, when he gets mistakenly drafted as a psychiatrist, he goes happily.

"When are you coming?" she stopped and asked.

"I can come tomorrow after the telecast. We'll work Sunday and Monday," I said, hopefully. She just sighed. I'm convinced people in the movie business like to string things out so it looks like they are really working.

By the time I sat down with Mimi to diagram the story, I had plenty of ideas and elements already written down. She had come up with enough information on U.S. Army regulations and procedures to give the story a spine, and in two days we put together one helluva yarn. What Mimi had found was that the Army had discarded all it had learned in World War II on treating combat fatigue and was handling cases in a totally different way now.

Previously psychiatrists tried to understand why the men were scarred by digging into their pasts. The catch-22 was anyone who wasn't scarred by Vietnam was crazy. The new method, the backbone of the story, was to take the patient to a front-line field hospital psych unit (*M.A.S.H.*?) and give them a one-course treatment of two weeks in a coma-like, thorazine-induced sleep, and when they woke up well-rested and clean, they found their combat gear and rifle on the end of the bed, with the psychiatrist reassuring them, "Don't worry. We'll make sure you don't let down your buddies. We'll be shipping you back to the front line soon." Yikes!

Into this mess comes Dr. Steiner, who has been mistakenly drafted into the Army from his holistic practice with the hippies of Haight-Ashbury in San Francisco. He becomes the psychiatrist in charge, and a hip male nurse lays out his course, telling him he can save many boys' lives by certifying they are loony and sending them back to the States. This inevitably results in his being court-martialed and dishonorably discharged, which is what he wants in the first place—to go home.

Our journey is to follow Steiner as he first becomes a doctor, then a psychiatrist, and finally a mature, responsible man. Along the way he falls in love (you have to have a love interest) with a Vietnamese maid who turns out to be a Vietcong commander.

Our comics are the patients, each with a unique story that spins from one laugh to another.

Our title is perfect: *Night Lights*. This was the answer to the question of what soldiers wanted most in their foxholes at night. They were all still pretty young, you know. Most of them had never been away from home.

In two days we had a solid script. Mimi was happy as hell. Leon loved it. I thought it would make a hell of a movie. We were talking

Dustin Hoffman and Richard Dreyfuss. We called King and made a date to meet him in New York at the end of the week.

This was the serendipitous beginning that turned me into a screenwriter, which is defined as someone who is paid to write a script. Making it into a movie was another thing entirely.

To Make a Movie

Mimi and I went to the plush offices of King & Hitzig Productions in New York, where we briefly met King's partner, a very nervous young man who had been in Vietnam.

"Very good first draft," Hitzig said, stuffing the papers in his briefcase and looking at his watch. "Gotta make a train."

He fled from us before we could say a word. Then King came out of his office, dressed the part of a movie producer in an elegant, well-cut suit, and brandishing a cigar the size of a baton.

"Have an H. Uppmann?" he asked, offering a humidor to Mimi and me, which we both declined.

"First off, I love the script," he remarked, puffing contentedly. "It will make a great movie. I'm talking Academy Awards here." Then suddenly he turned serious. "We got a major problem, though."

He fanned through the pages as Mimi and I shared a worried look.

"On page 71, we have the Vietnamese hooch maid talking to the other Vietnamese hooch maid in front of Steiner. They have to speak in Vietnamese, so how is the audience going to know what they are saying?"

I spoke up, "The same way those Indians on the high bridges over the Hudson are talking to the fucking dogs in your movie. How is the audience going to know what they are saying to the dogs? How are you solving that problem?"

I was almost laughing at King, because he was doing his best to sound like a real producer.

"It is a problem, I'll admit. We haven't whipped it yet."

"Subtitles?" Mimi ventured cautiously.

"I hate subtitles. Audiences can't read," King puffed.

"Voiceover in English?" she tried again.

"Doesn't work for me—two people talking at the same time."

"You'll think of something," I said reassuringly. "It isn't that vital to the script."

Happy to get rid of that, he put on his reading glasses, pursed his lips, and looked at me.

"On page 37, you have Hatrack the Schizo deliver a package to Steiner. Is it daylight?"

"It's the interior of an office. What difference does it make?"

"Well, if the office is lit by electric light, does Steiner turn off the light when he leaves?"

"No, he doesn't. He's mad at the Army and doesn't care how much energy he sucks up."

"Oh, good point. That fleshes out Steiner's character."

Mimi and I looked at each other. We had a long New York afternoon ahead of us and no way out, but King wanted to play producer, so we played. In the end, we were paid $100,000 for the script and Mimi was happy as she headed back to Los Angeles.

"Remember, that was the opening battle. We still have to fight the director, the star, and everybody else right down to the Vietnamese extras," she told me before boarding her flight.

"We'll see," I said, hurriedly banking my money and holding my breath until the check cleared. That is how I became a pinball in Hollywood's arcade game.

Eventually, when *Wolffen* died at the box office because the audience refused to believe Indians in Gotham talked to dogs, King & Hitzig Production Company put our script into *turnaround,* which is a clever euphemism for being one step away from dead in the water.

Poor Alan King died in 2004. He was a bright light in the entertainment field. He could do it all, and he did. With me, he was a great patient, responsive, obedient, and strong as an ox. He was bright as hell, as listening to his monologues prove. He tried hard as a movie producer, but that might have been just beyond his reach. One of the big things in his life was that he became the head of the Friars Club, his beloved club. I am a Friar, and that made me closer to Alan King. Oh, how he loved his Friars.

I'm proud to have been even a little part of his life in working with him in *Night Lights.* Had we made it with King as the producer, it would have been a big hit. His comedic sense would have made it so.

Then Alan Ladd, the big producer and son of a little star, got interested in the project, but Hollywood economics took a plunge and took Ladd and his company along with it, including our almost-certain-to-be-a-blockbuster. It went down for the second time.

Many years passed, and I had gotten over my disappointment at not seeing *Night Lights* made into a movie, when my son, Ferdie, came to see me. He had dreams of stardom and had been lucky enough to be an extra on the film, *Police Academy* (V, VI, VII, I can't remember), which was being shot in Miami. The producer/director of these highly successful comedies was Paul Mazlansky, and when he found out that Ferdie was actually the son of "The Fight Doctor," he asked him to bring me to the set.

Reluctantly, I went. I didn't care for his films, and I hated movie sets in general, but I found Mazlansky to be a terrific guy, a real man's man. I found out he played jazz on a flugel horn, and he loved boxing, so we really hit it off.

"I got a hell of a story I'd like to tell you," he said. "You're gonna love it." He asked if we could meet for dinner soon, and I agreed.

When we got together, I found my son had told him the history of *Night Lights,* and it interested him so much, he wanted to know more. Mazlansky became very animated when I spun the yarn and told him it was a finished, polished script, but was in turnaround at Warner Brothers.

Once again, serendipity floated *Night Lights* to the surface and threw it a lifebuoy, this time with a highly successful, moneymaking producer. He had clout, and he used it to buy the script from Warner Brothers for $40,000. We were back on dry land.

Mazlansky invited Mimi and me to his posh beach house in Malibu. When we arrived, we went out to his sundeck, where a tray of iced tea and a large bottle of sunscreen were waiting. I noticed a pair of high-powered binoculars hanging from Mazlansky's chair, which he immediately put to use. Every time a bikini-clad babe walked by on the beach below, Mazlansky would give her a close inspection with his X-ray vision goggles. This didn't sit well with Mimi, who was a conservative college professor and an ardent, if not strident, feminist. I surmised he was just prescreening for his next *Police Academy* film and told her so, but she was still rankled by his behavior, which didn't bode well for the work ahead.

Mazlansky finally sat down, picked up the dog-eared script, and dug right in.

"On page two, we need to punch up some one-liners."

I closed my eyes. "One-liners? The comedy in this script comes out of the characters and their situations, not from sitcom zingers."

"You need one-liners, believe me!" he insisted. "I have two guys who can really zest up this script."

Now I was rankled, right along with Mimi, but she spoke up first.

"This isn't written to be another tits and ass *Police Academy*," she said through her tightly clenched jaw. I looked at her, a bit surprised, but pleased.

"Well, we'll see," Mazlansky said, staring at a redhead with an incredible figure. To be honest, I wouldn't have minded having a pair of binoculars myself.

We worked our way through the script, each suggestion from Mazlansky driving a dagger deeper and deeper in our hearts. Our wonderful noir comedy was being turned into a matinee at Minsky's Burlesque House, with cheap, sleazy jokes.

Finally he came to our carefully scripted finish.

"There's not enough pizzaz!" he blurted. "What we need is a chase."

"A chase?" That really threw me. "We're in the middle of a Vietnam jungle!"

"We'll have 'em steal a cargo bus …" His eyes were lighting up like a Christmas parade. "And the 'Cong are running after them, when a chopper …"

"Oh God," I said, my eyes involuntarily rolling back into my head. I couldn't contain myself any longer. I was sure he had a hamster wheel inside his head in place of a brain. "That's awful."

I stood up, ready to leave all hope for *Night Lights* on Mazlansky's babe-watching perch, when he chimed in from behind his binoculars.

"Great afternoon of work, guys. It's Academy Award stuff, for sure. God, Dustin is going to flip." He stared hard at a Marilyn Monroe look-alike.

"Which one is Dustin going to play?" Mimi said sarcastically. "Bud Abbott or Lou Costello?"

I couldn't help but laugh at the inference, but it left Mazlansky with a streak over the top of his head.

Instead of enjoying the notoriety of an Academy Award, *Night Lights* was buried at sea when the studio offered Mazlansky two films to choose from. One was *Russia House,* which was to star Sean Connery and Michele Pfeiffer, to be directed by Hector Babenko, and to be filmed on location in Moscow with a very big budget. *Russia House* was a best-selling novel but turned out to be virtually unfilmable because the entire book was based on an old, over-the-hill British spy's running dialogue with himself. Mazlansky grabbed at it anyway, and *Night Lights* was dropped without another thought. I don't blame him. I suppose I would have done the same thing at the time, hindsight being what it is—20/20.

As it turned out, the Russian location shoot proved to be very difficult, the picture went over budget, it stunk, and it died an unmerciful death at the box office. There were no more Police Academies and no Academy Awards.

That is pretty much what happened with my first screenwriting venture. I didn't give up, though. I actually sold eight more scripts, one even made it to the big screen through an Italian producer, Salvatore Alabiso.

The moral of this story is just because you're introduced as a screenwriter at glitzy, star-studded parties doesn't mean you're anymore than a soggy clump at the bottom of the ocean. It's a good thing I didn't give up my day job as "The Fight Doctor."

✗✗✗✗✗✗

And that story that Mazlansky was so excited to tell me in the beginning? Well, it was this. Back in the early 1960s, Mazlansky was a broke and starving 40-year-old wannabe actor, hanging out at Cinecitta Studios in Rome, driving a cab, taking any part he could get. Most weeks he didn't have enough money left over to buy a stale cannoli. Sometimes he would tend bar at Dave's Dive in the Savoy Hotel, which was owned by Dave Crowley, a former European champion welterweight, who made his mark in the 1940s.

Crowley's place was very popular with the American movie crowd, and every time I came to Rome with the Muhammad Ali circus, as it was known, I would go there to unwind. Being Ali's physician got me a lot of attention and some great service there.

On September 10, 1966, Ali was scheduled to fight Karl Mildenburg in Frankfurt, Germany. Knowing how crazy Mazlansky was for Ali, Crowley surprised him by offering to take Mazlansky to the fight, sit in the first row, ringside, and, as a bonus, introduce him to me! Well, Mazlansky was beside himself with joy. I can't imagine why.

On fight night, they got there early to claim their prized seats, which had been given to Crowley to honor him for being a former champion. He was one of many former champs there that night, and all of them were introduced and asked to stand up while the crowd clapped and whooped in their honor.

Crowley's big moment finally came. He stood in the spotlight, filled with emotion, then started to choke, and promptly fell over with a heart attack. Mazlansky immediately ran for the phone, called for an ambulance, and they were whisked away to the hospital, where luckily, Crowley recuperated. But Mazlansky missed his golden opportunity to see Ali knock out Mildenberger (TKO 12), and he didn't meet me. Oh well, such is life.

That was the story he had been dying to tell me that was responsible for *Night Lights'* second resurrection.

But here's the real kicker. I wasn't even at Frankfurt for that fight. Angelo Dundee, the promoter I worked with, had another champion, Luis Manuel Rodriguez, in Madison Square Garden that same weekend, and because Angelo couldn't be there, he had sent me.

I didn't have the heart to tell Paul at the time—I figured I'd wait until the Academy Awards dinner. Pardon me if I couldn't wait any longer.

Jerry Lewis and the Cuban Revolution

Selling movie scripts is somewhat akin to hurricanes. There is a great flurry of activity, and as suddenly as it comes, it goes, leaving wreckage in its wake. Then, one day you see there is a hurricane warning. Again.

When we finished our travails with *Night Lights,* and it dawned on us that the project was dead as a doornail, we fell back to rest. Where had we gone wrong?

The most obvious thing was we failed to attach a star. With a star signed, we would be halfway home. A director signed was good too, but a *star* was the thing.

During my years recording the wild escapades of the Cuban immigrants I had collected some wildly funny tales, but none as hilarious as that of two cousins, Flaco (the thin one) and Baby. To whet your appetite, let me tell you their method of escape was to steal a Russian motor torpedo boat on Christmas Eve. It goes without saying neither man was a sea-faring man. Hooked yet?

As usual I was involved in many other activities, and one in particular netted me a producing partner, who, as it turned out, could attach a star, a *major star.*

Sherry Reinker was a tall, vivacious, beautiful blonde. She'd been a prize athlete, a baton-twirling champion, a beauty queen, and a driven competitor. At the time I met her she had invented an event, which was

named the Bravo Latin Music Awards. To get the job done she needed
a Hispanic partner, a good showbiz lawyer, and a whole load of prayers.

It was a long hard haul, but in 1987 she put together a glittering
show in Santo Domingo. It was a scintillating night. She flew home to
Miami, assured of a major source of income for the life of the show. At
least, that is what she thought.

By the time the wolves picked over the skeleton of the contract, she
found she owned nothing. Lawsuit time. Agony. Angst. Enter Ferdie
Pacheco and a funny Hispanic film script.

She read it as a novel, *Only in America,* and she phoned right away.
"This is one for Jerry Lewis."

She and Lewis had been friends and had almost married. They were
still close.

I said, "Send it!"

She did. Lewis read it and phoned immediately.

"There are at least five movies in this book. It's hilarious. The best
I've read in years. Come see me, let's talk."

We jumped on a plane and met Mr. Showbiz in his offices. They
were in a mall in a storefront. My heart sank.

Through the years I'd been on the fringes of the Lewis tornado.
Sometimes he was gracious and mannerly. Sometimes, notoriously
irreverent, an enfant terrible. Sometimes crude, vicious, and hurtful. I
approached him as if he were a Croatian minefield. I'd lay back and let
the personable Reinker do the talking.

Lewis was the soul of kindness. He knew of me through Ali, and
my TV work.

Lewis was a sick man, but he hid his various infirmities very well,
and he looked about five years younger than his age. On this day he was
very flattering, going over many of the highlights of the novel and
showing how he would make them funnier. No doubt about it, the key
part was Popoff, the Jewish liability insurance case lawyer, a devious,
crafty con-artist and a man without a conscience but with a heart of
gold in the end. ("I gotta think about my kids. They can't see me in a
bad light.")

After an hour of laughing, we settled down to cutting up the deal.
Reinker and I would produce. With Lewis, of course. Lewis would co-
write the script with me, of course. And, ahem, Lewis would star, as
well, of course.

While this was going on, my mind turned on to caution. I'd been
around the bad Jerry Lewis, and I remember two of the sightings par-

ticularly well. In the first, Lewis was due to star with Milton Berle for a weekend at the Deauville in Miami Beach. I had become friendly with a top ex-agent, Vic Jarmel, who knew everyone in showbiz and who was the man to look up in South Miami. On this afternoon we went to pick up Berle, and he was steaming. Lewis had pulled rank to finish the show. Berle would open for Jerry. Because both were mammoth egos, it figured to be a deal breaker. But both needed the work, so Berle backed down reluctantly.

When he got in the car, steam was coming out of his ears and his eyes narrowed.

"The little fuck is in for a showbiz lesson. I'll open all right. Jerry is doing my act anyway. I'll go back and do all my routines—only I'll pull out all stops. I'll show the audience how these routines should really be done."

At rehearsals, Berle made detailed notes of what Lewis was going to do. Lewis was flattered that Berle was that interested in his part of the show.

That opening night Berle was so sensational that he got several standing ovations and a roaring ovation good-bye at the end of his end of the show.

Lewis sat in amazement. Berle had just done his act. He was holding a gun with no bullets to shoot. Lewis was dead in the water. The audience was reserved and respectful, but the laughs were few and far between, and there were long stretches of silence. Lewis sang a bad imitation of Jolson, he danced a flaccid imitation of Sammy Davis Jr., and his little bad-boy misbehaving act had worn out, and his 50-year-old face could not bring it off. It must have been the worst night of his life. Berle was beaming.

The other Lewis experience was when he came to Miami to bring a movie company to make another Lewis film. It didn't get off the ground, but he left a $1 million dollar debt in Miami. He left a load of angry creditors and trades people.

Both of those experiences were fresh in my mind. I said nothing to Reinker, who was bubbling in happiness. On the way back Reinker started making plans to raise $400,000 as start-up money to provide a working script and pay Lewis's expenses.

Reinker was a successful publicist, operating nine magazines from the big social clubs, Palm Bay Club, Cricket, and Jockey Club. She knew how to tout the Miami social set. She knew party people, the people who could drop $1 million on a movie without crying in their gazpacho.

The group that the energetic, industrious Reinker put together was a group of successful millionaires who met once a month at Williams Island to entertain deals. They were 14 in number. They were young— a plastic surgeon, a Toyota dealer, and lawyers, and a few other retired millionaires. The called themselves "The Jews" because they *were*.

As soon as Reinker dropped the Lewis name, they started salivating and reminiscing about when they had seen Martin and Lewis.

Of course, we had a letter of commitment from Lewis. They all agreed $400,000 was a drop in the bucket. But then it hit; for that kind of money, they want to see Lewis in person.

"But can you get him here for next month's meeting? We'd like to hear his plans for the film."

Well, folks, I did not want to pay for tickets to bring Lewis, his Caddy-chauffeur, wife, and dog, to and from California. Neither did Reinker.

Surprise! Surprise! Lewis said he would pay, but wanted a compromise—a luxury apartment on the golf course—all of the perks, of course. The Jews said, "Of course."

The meeting got off to a riotous start. After all of the handshaking, signing of eight by 10s and reminisces about Atlantic City in 1948, we got down to our formal meeting.

"Gentlemen, I'll not lie to you. I'm *not* here to pick up a niggardly $400,000. I can get that on any street corner in Beverly Hills.

"What I want to see is an $8 million commitment to make the film. This is the freshest, funniest material I have seen in 20 years. With Miami as the backdrop and the Cuban population here, what we got is a socko-boffo comedy hit."

The 14 Jews scrunched down as if they had been hit over the head by pile drivers. The first to speak was an 80-year-old investor with a white beard. I called him "The Lion of Judea," and I recognized in him the end to our project.

"Mr. Lewis, when we finish this masterpiece, where will you sell it? You don't have studio backing now, do you? Who will distribute our pearl of a film?"

Lewis nodded all through the question as if he had anticipated the question and had the right answer on the palm of his hand.

"Ha, ha!" said Lewis, shaking his finger at "The Lion of Judea." "I knew you'd be the one to bring that up; ha, ha, you ol' mumser you." He actually tweaked the old man's cheek.

The old man held him in a steely stare. "So?"

"Listen, I'll take these reels to four major studios who have been begging for a new Jerry Lewis film. I make family movies, Mister, clean things you can take your kids to. Studios want to pay and distribute our film. No problema! What we'll have is a bidding war!"

"For our money, what percentage return do we get? How long before we see a profit? How about other residuals? Tape? Foreign sales? The Greek maritime fleet?"

"Whoa, whoa. You guys are always ahead of the game. I haven't decided who I'm going to let put up the money. Those are legal questions. I'll send my lawyer to talk to you."

"Mr. Lewis," "The Lion of Judea" rumbled deeply. "When is the last time you made a movie in America?"

"Seventeen years, but I was working in France, where I am considered a genius and have received the Legion of Honor."

"And when is the last time you made a film in France?" "The Lion of Judea" was relentless.

"Fourteen years, but that's because of internal European friction and politics," Lewis said in a rather unconvincing manner. I could feel the air leaving our balloon.

"Hmmm. When can we see this lawyer?"

"Next month when you next meet," said Lewis as if he had just won the Super Bowl. He went to the bar with us filled with optimism.

"There. That was easy. I got 'em eating out of the palm of my hand."

I looked at Reinker. Even the ever-optimistic happy-go-lucky Reinker had tears in her eyes.

"Well, we came close," she said simply.

Next month arrived too soon for my taste. Not a word from Lewis, except that he was sending his killer closer Beverly Hills lawyer to rub out "The Lion of Judea."

When the attorney called with the landing information, he said he'd make his own arrangements with a limo. Thank you.

When would we meet to discuss our battle plan? Not necessary, he'd talked to Lewis. He'd be at the Fontainebleau, at his suite making calls. Our meeting was for 7:30 p.m. since we were to sit down with the Jews at 8 p.m. Little time to talk.

"Not to worry," he says airily.

I called Reinker.

"Worst possible news, Sherry, we've got a Jewish entertainment attorney from Beverly Hills, and his name is Dale Yorkshire."

"As in the pudding," says Reinker, laughing.

"You got it."

At 7:30 p.m. exactly on the nose, Dale Yorkshire, the Earl of Beverly Hills, strode in looking like a clone of George Hamilton, smiled his 100-tooth gleaming white smile, and put out his delicate hand.

"Hi."

He brought forth what can only be described as the second coming of the 18-year-old Lana Turner.

"Hi," she says in a Marilyn whisper, "I'm Dale's—secretary."

I got the feeling she was suppressing a laugh.

"The Lion of Judea" ain't happy. We ate lavishly at these meetings, which was too much for him. Reinker, Yorkshire, Mona (for that was her name), and I were far too much tariff to bear.

As the meal progressed, Yorkshire and Mona were engaged in a lot of under the table hanky panky, and a lot of above the table hand play. We didn't share many thoughts. He seemed sublimely confident.

The time for his presentation was here. He got up slowly, like Churchill about to address the House of Commons.

"Gentlemen, Mr. Lewis has told me of the gem of a movie he wants to make. He feels it will top the *Bellboy* or the *Professor* movies. He has asked for $8 million, more or less, for we know he has a penchant for going over budget."

There was a groan from the 14 Jews.

He brought all kinds of charts with him—pie charts, bar charts, and charts of the harbor of New Orleans. He spouted percentages and indecipherable gobbly gook. It's double talk, La La Land bullshit. Most of the Jews ware car dealers. You weren't going to out-bullshit a guy that sells Toyotas for God's sake.

There was a moment of stunned silence, Yorkshire looked confident, as if waiting for the 14 Jews to spring forward with checks adding up to $8 million. Mona looked proud, her hand squeezing his calf.

"Questions?"

"Mister Lewis, when he was here stated that four major studios, MGM, Warners, Columbia, and Universal, are dying to get into a bidding war to buy the finished film. Is this, in fact, so?"

Charming Yorkshire let a smile of condescension flit across his face. His delicate hand, slowly pulled off his Porsche sunglasses, his eyes, a beautiful blue, crinkled in a Meg Ryan smile. He began to laugh slowly at first and then in a loud bark.

"Did Jerry *actually* say that? Oh God. Actors. They never know when to quit with the bullshit. What did he say? Four. Four major studios? After Jerry Lewis? Christ, he can't get in the gate at most of those studios."

"No, no. We are out here as an indie production, and we'll make our own distribution deal based on Jerry's huge popularity in America."

"And the percentages he quoted?"

"Figment of a blown out of proportion ego."

I tugged at his pants. I kicked his shin.

"Are you for us or against us?" I felt like I was in the final scenes of *The Exorcist,* watching this Hollywood dandy turn green and red-eyed with his head swiveling in his Brooks Brothers sport coat and about to vomit oatmeal on Reinker and me. I knew we were doomed. Even the Toyota dealer had seen enough.

"We'll call you," he said to Reinker with a nice smile of pity as if seeing her off on a train to Dachau.

"There's one thing worse than an actor in a film deal, and that is an actor's lawyer," Reinker said, crestfallen.

"You'll learn," said "The Lion of Judea," patting me kindly on the shoulder.

We never came close with that deal, although of all my scripts, this story was far and away the best, and to put the dagger in my heart, Lewis would have been brilliant as the mad but irresistibly loveable Popoff.

CHAPTER 15

Winds of Change

One of the things that is permanent in the makeup of network television is change; change for the better, change for the worse, and change for the hell of it.

We had gone a pretty long way, about four years, with our laissez-faire method of doing boxing when the winds of change blew our way. It was a shame, because we were on a roll.

We were still under the benevolent guidance of Watson, but the powers that be dictated that we shape up the winning team. Some would get promoted upward (like Weisman to executive producer). Some were fired, and some new faces were placed in the executive ranks to impose order on anarchy (Sean McManus, Bert Zeldin, and Ken Schanzer).

My happy little world of boxing began to cave in with the punishment of Mr. Inside, Mike I. Cohen. Cohen, a blustery New Yorker, liked the rough-and-tumble world of sports. He was a goalie at heart. Matthew McCarthy, Linda Johnson's assistant in the *Sportsworld* family, was shy, diffident, sensitive, laid back, and very intelligent. The two rubbed each other the wrong way. Sparks flew when they passed each other in the hallway, and a confrontation was inevitable.

One fine day they had a shouting match. McCarthy had a sharp tongue and goaded Cohen until his only recourse was a stiff right cross to the mouth. One punch and it was a knock out. Cohen won the battle but lost the war.

NBC had a ruling: No physical violence. Watson had adopted Cohen, warts and all, and depended on his rough opinions. He didn't want to fire him, so he kept him at a highly reduced position. For example, he no longer came to fights with me. That was a terrible loss for me, because Cohen loved boxing and boxing people and was a huge help in every department. My heart broke to see him relegated to nothing better than an office boy.

But after every storm, the sun shines. The next fight after the banishment, Cohen introduced me to Kevin Monaghan, a handsome, quiet Irish kid. He became my shadow and partner for my final years at NBC, and I grew to think of him as a son, or at the very least, a younger brother.

O Kevin-Me-Boy

Kevin Monaghan came on without fanfare or introduction. One day he wasn't there, the next day he was. Cohen, normally a fountain of information, had not told me of his own demotion, nor of the hiring of Monaghan to slowly take over Cohen's duties. With Cohen out, it meant our most excellent Mr. Inside–Mr. Outside method of getting fights approved was out. Because I was still in control of making NBC fights, what did I have to do to okay a contract? It sort of went through McManus and Zeldin, but everybody seemed to have an opinion. One day I saw a copy of *Ring* magazine in Jeff "Bad News" Coker's office. Coker was fresh out of law school and did the boxing contracts. It was a mess. It was very important to know that the deal I gave my word on to boxing promoters would be honored. All of my perceived power lay in the strength of my word. If I didn't have that, I had nothing.

If I was momentarily depressed at the loss of my bullyboy defender, it took no time at all to realize that he had replaced himself with a jewel of a guy. Even in the end, Cohen was looking out for me when he brought in Monaghan as his understudy.

Monaghan looked like he was out of a 1930s Irish IRA play. He looked pure Dublin. Not that he had an Irish accent; he didn't. It's just that he stepped out of a James Joyce novel, a Sean O'Casey play. Boy, was he Irish.

Monaghan was not shy, but he was very quiet. He didn't initiate conversation, and he listened intently to everything that was said and managed to respond appropriately. He looked very serious, but he had a sparkling Irish wit, and he loved characters, like I did. And he enjoyed listening to my long stories about the old days of boxing at the Fifth Street Gym and my Mafia stories about Ybor City. In short, he was a windbag's dream; he was a good listener. What a pair we were—a talker and a listener—a marriage made in heaven.

Monaghan did not have Cohen's love or knowledge of boxing, but he was a bright lad, and before long he became a part of me. It was as if I had imparted my lifetime of boxing knowledge and love into Monaghan by sheer dint of sitting next to me on the long limo rides to Atlantic City, and by osmosis he became as good as I in making matches. I was delighted, because I loved calling the fights with Albert, but with the roadblocks and interference from Schanzer and his puppy dog wannabe Coker, I was getting gray-headed and hypertensive. I hated making fights. Two bouts in particular spelled my end as a matchmaker.

Barry McGuigen and the Luck O' the Irish.

We had developed and shown a great Irish kid, Barry McGuigen, whose father sang "Danny Boy" before each fight. The din of Dublin, or Belfast, was unbelievable. McGuigen won his fights before the first bell rang. A McGuigen fight was a television delight.

What McGuigen could not accomplish was to fight for the championship in Ireland. Eusebio Pedrosa was a legendary Hispanic champ who had held the title for so long that no one in Panama could remember who had been champ before him.

NBC needed a big fight for May sweeps month when we had real cash to spend. Watson was a dyed-in-the-wool Irishman. He loved McGuigen as if he were his own son. I told him that through my Latin underground, and with a little trickery—which was best he didn't know about—I could possibly make a McGuigen–Pedrosa fight in Ireland for the title. Impossible, the boxing fraternity said. Not in *this century.*

It so happened I knew Pedrosa's manager was coming to Miami. We were old-time friends. We had Roberto Duran in common. He felt like I was an honorary Panamanian. We met at my house. My beautiful wife, a gourmet cook, laid out a spread. He loved my art, offering to buy one. And when all was rosy, I popped the question. May … Ireland … title fight … McGuigen … how much? That was the only question unanswered.

I was amazed to hear that I could make the match for $225,000 (for both fighters). Remember, these were different days. It was a fair price, on the high side for TV.

I knew McGuigen would accept anything, so I made the match in my house. I couldn't wait to tell Watson. I called him at home, and he did his version of an Irish jig. Boy, oh boy. McGuigen versus Pedrosa in Ireland in sweeps month. What a coup!

Then the vicious, malignant dogs began to pick it apart. "What if …" began every objection from the dogs. Even Watson began to weaken. Only Monaghan held firm and was my voice in the meetings. Monaghan fought hard to keep McGuigen–Pedrosa on our May schedule.

To wrap this up, NBC did not do the McGuigen–Pedrosa fight. ABC did. I wanted to go home and puke. I went all of the way to London to see the fight I had made. McGuigen won the title in a hard, hard fight.

I stood at the doorway of a packed dressing room, enjoying the hysterical cheering of the crowd. Suddenly McGuigen called the crowd to be quiet. The room fell silent.

"There in the back doorway is the man I owe this championship to, Dr. Pacheco of NBC." And he came forth to hug me.

Well, I didn't get to do the fight, but I got to have a defining moment. It was almost worth it.

I knew I had to get out of matchmaking. As Schanzer had said, I was trying too hard, and I hated to lose too much. I hate to admit it, but he was right. He didn't mind losing the fight of the year because he hated boxing. It was the main difference I had with him; I loved boxing, he hated it.

✗✗✗✗✗✗✗

Schanzer's meddling in boxing just plain made no sense. Here is one instance of that. One day he came up with a Schanzer Rule for Economizing in boxing. If I agreed with a promoter that we would buy his event for $150,000, I should bring it to NBC, where they would reduce it by $50,000. This was a flat $50,000 applied to all contracts. Huh? Suppose I made a fight for $50,000, then what?

No amount of arguing could change his mind, so I came up with an Ybor City solution, very sociopathic. I took a fight I had made with Russell Peltz for $100,000 and a handshake and I instructed him to send it to NBC for $150,000. Schanzer gleefully cut it to look right, and we were all happy. I did this many times until he relented or caught on, I don't know which, and it didn't matter; he was wrong.

Schanzer insisted on coming to the Olympics in Los Angeles with Watson and then-president of NBC Jack Welch, who really knew boxing. I didn't want to go. What for? Watson, under the influence of Schanzer, had turned down the buy of the century. Lou Duva, my faithful friend, offered me two bright shining stars, Pernell Whitaker and Meldrick Taylor, for a thin $60,000, provided they both won the gold medal.

Of course, Schanzer's network nitwits were slavering over Mark Breland, a skinny flyweight who had more than 300 amateur fights and was certain to wear out in the pros. Our ignorant colleagues at ABC were offering $1 million. Unbelievably Schanzer wanted to try to top ABC! And they turned down Taylor and Whitaker for $60,000 and a two-year exclusive contract!

Here's a look at how infantile Schanzer could get. Watson insisted Zeldin be my new know-nothing keeper and I come to Los Angeles.

"For what?" I said, mad as hell. "You already got the brains of boxing there."

He was adamant; I had to come.

The first night we ran into a nice humiliation. No one had thought to get us credentials! They did have upper-deck tickets, sitting with the Yugoslav soccer team. I wanted to catch the next plane home, but Zeldin restrained me.

"Tomorrow we'll get credentials," said the patient company man.

Next morning was no different. I confronted Watson; he expressed surprise and dismay but got in his limo with Schanzer and left us behind. But not before I made him a bet.

"I'll bet you $10 I'll be sitting beside Howard Cosell at the ABC position before you are comfortable in your public ringside seats."

He smiled. "You're on!"

I showed up without any credentials or seats. Security was tough. I went to a gate where a young, good-looking black athlete was taking tickets. He recognized me immediately.

"The Fight Doctor!" he said, asking me for an autograph, which I happily gave him as I pitched my story.

"Hey, I left all of my credentials in the hotel room. I got to get ringside to report this fight—get me through."

And so, through a series of boxing fan ushers, I was seated beside the ABC position before Welch and Watson took their seats. I waved at Welch and pointed to a $10 bill for Watson. This turned out to be the seating arrangement for the entire dreary Olympics. That proved I am more boxing than television, once again.

When it was over, we had a meeting in the lobby. Welch, knowledgeable as hell about boxing talent, said, "The best talent here is Pernell Whitaker and Meldrick Taylor. Future champs. We could have had them for $60,000, but these chumps passed."

"The best talent in the Olympics is a flyweight," Schanzer insisted.

We all groaned at his obstinate stupidity. That's the thing about lobbyists, even when they are obviously wrong, they still stick to their guns. It's practice, I guess.

"And what do we do with a 106-pound man on NBC boxing? Match him with a tiny guy from Siam, Japan, the Philippines? What can we do with a guy that tiny? Make a paperweight out of him?"

I couldn't believe his dogged wrong-headedness in front of his boss. Case closed. Everyone got back into the limos, sulking about the thin boxer who got away to ABC.

Postscript: Breland didn't last more than a year before he fell apart. The flyweight suffered a career-ending injury and did not have a pro career. So much for the Olympics. We had a chance at a major coup and instead, we got skunked. I had to get out of there!

One Last Schanzer Story: The Sly Try

One day when I was on my way to see Watson, I noted that there was no one in the offices. Schanzer, Coker, McManus, Zeldin, and the whole boxing cabal were gone. Smelling a rat, I went to Watson, who was also gone. The secretary, looking surprised, said to me, "They're all down in the conference room having a meeting with Sylvester Stallone."

Sly! Here in the executive offices! This was just what I agreed with Ohlmeyer wouldn't happen. If you won't allow King, Arum, Peltz, or Duva to come pitch their product, why make an exception for Sly? Guess.

I had had a series of dealings with Stallone, all revealing that he had the best of intentions, deep pockets, and a sucker's gullible mind for con games. Once we had his heavyweight against Lou Duva's Scott Frank to be fought on Sunday in Studio 1A in the NBC building with all of the casts of Broadway shows invited free. Sly lost control of his heavyweight when John Derek offered him the fighter role of Tarzan opposite his wife, Bo Derek. The first shot was the big lug running down the beach in a loincloth. John Derek was shocked to notice that Tarzan's tits were bigger than Bo's, so they put him on the first slow freighter out. End of Tarzan; end of TV fight.

The fight never took place. Now Sly was back pitching a con to NBC, and the network nitwits lined up to drool over a movie star. This is exactly what I had in mind when I agreed with Ohlmeyer that it would not happen. Well, Ohlmeyer was gone, and the lobbyist was here, along with Stallone.

I walked in, steam coming out of my ears, and found a smiling Sly. Seated with him was Larry Holmes's trainer, Rich Giachetti, an ex-racket guy who dabbled in promoting and managing fighters.

"Hiya, Richie, does the parole board know you're traveling out of state?" I said. Richie and I are close pals. He knows I know he's a con. "You look just like your pictures in the post office."

"Go easy, Doc," he whispered as I passed by. Sly waved happily. The nitwits looked guilty.

"Whatcha got?" I said to him, taking my place.

"We propose to go to every nook and cranny of the country and find heavyweights who have talent but have slipped through the cracks of the boxing promoters, and we'll have an elimination tournament exclusively on NBC!"

I looked at Giachetti with a fisheye. He looked sheepish. That is one of the oldest cons in boxing, and Sly, who made a fortune drama-tizing the con in his endless *Rocky* series, had bought into it as well. Actors! They really get to believe their scripts are real.

With as much kindness as I could muster, I shot this down. I didn't want to knock Giachetti, whom I liked a lot, out of his gig with the gullible actor. Fact: There are *no* unknown heavyweights in the country. *Tough Man competitions cover amateurs who like to beat the stuffing out of other amateurs.* Once they get in the ring with a real boxer, it is tantamount to murder.

"Well, what would you say if I told you we had the best-kept secret in boxing, the next Middleweight Champion of the World, who already has a 60-4 record in the pros?"

Stallone, looking spiffy in a cream-colored three-piece suit, flashed his million-dollar smile.

"Oh my God, Richie, don't tell me you stuck him with Vinnie Curto?"

Giachetti looked guilty; Sly looked surprised.

"I'll tell you what, Sly, Vinnie will string you out until he's into you for 50 Gs, then he'll break your heart. You'd do better to put Vinnie in your movies. He's a good actor," I said as Sly looked stunned.

Angelo Dundee and Murray Gaby had had Curto at 30-0, and Angelo had decided to make his move. We had put him in with Rodrigo Valdez and Tony Licatta in New Orleans, a couple of top-ranked Philly lions, and three other fighters, and Curto had lost four and tied one. He had fought bravely and fought like hell, but from that point on, Curto decided that he would avoid pain at all costs. And because he was a great runner, his fights took on the aspects of a track meet. He was interested in boxing as an investment, not a career.

"Sly, $50,000 or a career in movies, and then he moves on."

Sly was looking unnerved. The meeting was over. Giachetti was out of suggestions; Sly was beaten by truth and reality. I felt sorry for him; he wanted to be in the real world of boxing so bad, but the script was just not right.

The Holmes Fiasco: Farewell to All That

McManus was reading an old copy of *Ring* magazine when he got a bright idea. Someone had suggested a Holmes–Frazier fight. Being totally ill-informed about boxing and being a network nitwit in training, he naturally assumed that Holmes–Frazier would be a blockbuster ratings winner. Quietly I took him off to the side when he suggested I go out and make the fight.

"Frazier? That would have been a good fight 10 years ago. Joe Frazier? He's gone, shot, retired. This Frazier is his son, Marvis. The only similarity between the two is how they spell their last name. Joe? Yes. Marvin? No."

Marvis was nothing like Joe. He had had 10 protected fights, which hardly qualified him as an opponent for a great champ like Larry Holmes.

Lost in his reverie, McManus didn't seem to get it. I hurried over to Watson's office and made my pitch. Watson always smiled when I told him of McManus's infantile daydreams. It was as if he was McManus's doting father.

"Don't ever think of making that fight. If there is any mercy, the boxing board shouldn't license it."

Watson laughed and said, "Don't worry."

Right then, I knew I should worry.

Months later Watson called me in Miami to say he had a window of opportunity for a primetime fight on Thanksgiving weekend. He wanted a blockbuster, a big-name fight, like, say, Holmes–Frazier! Huh?

I exploded into 10 minutes of screaming. Watson heard me out, and when I finished, he said, "Do me a favor. Get Holmes–Frazier. I told the network we could do it. I'm asking you to get me out of a tight spot. Do it for me. Make the match. You got $1 million."

There it was. Watson had been aces-up for me. He had backed me in everything I wanted to do. He stood up to King-Arum-Sulamain and all of the corrupt boxing people, and I owed him. I started having nonsense conversations with him.

"We're paying Holmes $1 million. What are we paying Frazier?"

"I gave you $1 million," he said.

"Which we paid Holmes," I explained patiently.

"You figure it out. I gave you $1 million."

As if somehow I could do a mathematical jujitsu and come out with two top-name fighters for $1 million, I just let that lay on the table until they came to the obvious answer. They needed a bit more for Marvis, and we got it.

I had assured Watson many times that the fight wouldn't last four rounds if we were lucky, based on the fact that statistically Holmes had never knocked anyone out after the fourth. That, and the fact that he loved Joe Frazier and might be kind to Marvis out of respect for Joe, and just beat the shit out of Marvis for four rounds. Meanwhile, we had a two-hour show to do. What would fill the void?

"Get me a good co-feature championship bout with a name fighter."

"Okay. How much dough do we have?"

"I gave you $1 million already, and some extra for Marvis," he said in a pained voice as if I was asking him for a personal loan.

"Look Art, I just sold you my antique Packard for a million bucks. Now, you come back and want to buy my 1947 Cadillac convertible that costs $50,000 more. And you say, 'I just gave you a million for the Packard.' What do you think I'd say?"

"We haven't got any more money."

"And we don't have a name championship fight—and two long hours on primetime with nothing to put on."

"Who could you get?" he said, weakening.

"'Boom Boom' Mancini," I dropped the good news.

"Fighting whom?"

"Depends on the money you give me."

"What? I already gave you $1 million!"

"That again! Wake up and come to the party. We spent that million and then some."

"Well, that's all we got," he said stubbornly, as if I should solve the problem of getting a big attraction like "Boom Boom" to fight for NBC on primetime for free!

Are you beginning to see why I started looking for a way to get out of making fights? My blood pressure started to rise, I couldn't sleep at night, trying to make sense of this insanity, and somehow I knew it would get worse. Schanzer and his twisted mind lay in wait.

Somehow I pierced Watson's insane obstinacy, and he came up with a paltry fee for Mancini. I promised Mancini a truly easy fight.

"Who is he going to fight? I hope it's a worthwhile challenger, who'll give him a tough fight and give us rounds." I heard the voice of Schanzer the agitator in the background.

"Depends on how much money we got," I said patiently, knowing now that I would have to again go through the insanity of the paucity of purse act with Watson.

"What? I just gave you a load of cash for 'Boom Boom.' That's what you have."

"For 'Boom Boom.' Now, what about his opponent?"

After a few weeks of Mickey Mouse wheeling, Watson came up with $10,000 for the opponent. For that type of chump change, no worthy opponent would step into our NBC primetime Thanksgiving extravaganza and be knocked out! Not likely.

I had just seen an insanely brave Cuban kid named Johnny Torres take a savage beating for 10 rounds in Miami and lose a close decision. Man, could he take a punch! I got him to sign. He needed the bread. When would he ever be featured on a primetime fight so all America could see him?

Watson took a vacation up in Canada, hunting elk, or Eskimos, or whatever it is that fat, Jack Daniels-soaked executives do in frigid Canada. He couldn't be reached. But before he left, he called me, semi-apologetic.

"I know you don't want this fight, but I gotta have it. My ass is on the line to produce, and a heavyweight title fight on Thanksgiving gets me off the hook. I know it's been tough, but make sure nothing goes wrong. I gotta have this fight. Promise me you'll do everything in your power to hold it together."

Who could say no to that? I couldn't. I was between a rock and a hard place. The easiest way out was to let the whole fight fall apart on its own. The Holmes fight was a joke. Marvis? For God's sake, this wasn't a fight, it was an execution. Shame on me, a proponent of boxing safety, an opponent of blatant mismatches, fighting hard as hell to keep this farce together. Similarly, Mancini mugging this poor little Cuban exile was nothing to look forward to. Yet, Watson was in a spot, and he had asked me directly to promise to hold it together, to "save him," whatever that meant.

With Watson gone, Schanzer arose from the shadows of the hallway and began his vitriolic fight to sink the bout. I tried to tell him

Watson had ordered me directly to make sure we filled the date. One day in the midst of a fierce phone fight, Schanzer yelled at me, "You don't understand. When Arthur Watson is not here, *I* am NBC."

What bombast. What bullshit. It was all I could do to laugh at this pathetic egomaniac.

Patiently I said, "Go look at your door. See the nameplate. It has screws holding it in place. One day an NBC workman will come and unscrew that plate, and you'll be history, just like Jeff Mason before you. Here is the hard fact; you're not Arthur Watson, much as you'd like to be. When Watson calls and tells me to jettison the fight, I'll gladly do so and breathe a sigh of relief."

Schanzer got so determined to win that he got to the point where he accused me of fighting so hard to save the fight because my contract called for a $10,000 bonus for every primetime fight. Fortunately, the reason I was so independent in my thought and action was that I had a healthy bank balance and had what people in the entertainment business call *fuck you money*. Schanzer couldn't fight that.

Anyway, despite a nasty running battle with the Black Knight, we managed to have the fight. In two hours of TV programming we had to show two rounds of fighting, six minutes. Not even Mike Weisman, the magician, could save us. We looked like fools. It looked like this was my idea. King and Arum, the New York press, and my enemies in boxing did a victory dance. They thought I'd be fired. None knew this was Watson's turd. And naturally, Watson wasn't defending me and wasn't about to claim the disaster as his own.

What happened was a tragic comedy of errors. Holmes was perfectly happy to carry Frazier for four or six rounds as a gesture of respect to the old man. But some goofus put their dressing rooms next to each other. As Holmes lay still to take his nap, he began hearing a pep rally going on next door, with drums, bongos, and tribal chanting, the main gist of which was, "Kill the motherfucker! Knock out Holmes!"

Holmes, normally a mild-mannered man who fights dispassionately, worked up a head of steam. He came into the ring with fire in his eyes. He stormed out at the bell and overwhelmed a badly outclassed kid. Knockout in one!

Weisman played the knockout over and over from every angle; we interviewed the world and still we had a lot of program to fill. Now it was up to Mancini to show a quality of mercy and stretch out his fight.

While we were filling with crap, I ran to talk to Mancini. I was now in a desperate position. I had to do something dangerous, which I had never done in 30 years of boxing.

"'Boom Boom,' I gotta ask a favor. You know we are in a big jam with time. Now I got you an easy little kid from Miami. You always knock out these tomato cans in one round, so the audience never really gets to see how good a boxer you are.

"Do you think you could box pretty for about six or seven rounds? I mean, if this kid turns dangerous, knock him out, but he's coming off a big beating, so don't hurt him, okay?"

I felt like hell. I'd never asked any fighter to carry anyone. Boxing is a dangerous game. This kid could surprise Mancini, but Mancini was the champ, head and shoulders above this poor little immigrant Cuban kid. If Mancini cracked to the press that I asked him to carry the kid, I would be finished. I felt awful.

"Okay, Doc, no problem," said Mancini, giving me his wonderful reassuring smile. "I'll just have fun for a few rounds."

I went back to my broadcast position and never said a word to Albert or to Weisman. I wasn't going to advertise that I was interfering with the conduct of a fight. I don't mean I was suicidal. I knew how easy the kid was, how little a threat he was to Mancini. If we could get seven rounds, I'd sleep well that night.

We stretched the entrance of the fighters and the introduction, and as I remember, Weisman went low enough to re-rack the Duk Koo Kim death at the hands of Mancini. Finally we ran out of any possible reason to stretch anymore, and the fight began.

The first two punches told me we were in trouble. A stiff left jab popped Torres's head back and then a sizzling right cross established Mancini's evil intentions. The knockout came with a minute left in the *first round!* Mancini attacked Torres as if Torres had just stolen Mancini's mother's handbag. It was brutal and fast. When I had to interview him and reminded him of our conversation, he said, "I thought you were kidding," and manfully, I said, "I was."

The final act of this tragic comedy farce came when we had a gathering of the dog pound in Watson's office later that week. Semi-officially, it was called to burn me at the stake.

It was a foggy day, the kind of day that blotted out the neighboring skyscrapers. Watson had his high-backed chair turned to stare at the clouds, as if he had nothing to do with the proceedings.

After a bit of desultory small arms firing, Schanzer, the leader of the mad dogs, opened up on me. I cut him off by directing my comments to Watson.

"Arthur, turn that chair around and face the music. Tell these yowling dogs whose idea this fight was, who ordered it, who had to have this fight happen. It's bad enough I'm taking the heat for this in the press and on the street, but I'm not taking the fall for this in the office."

That was basically the end of that. Watson kind of took the fall and kind of admitted he ordered me to get the fight and get it done. And that, as they say, was that. Case closed. For all intents and purposes that ended my days as a matchmaker. Oh, we sputtered for a while, but Watson had his eye on Monaghan as my replacement, and I was thrilled to death.

Having Monaghan there saved my on-camera job, because I knew he would do as good a job as I, and he wouldn't cave in to Arum and King. I could do the commentary stuff in cruise control. My blood pressure would come back to normal. I would not have stayed if the matchmaking fell in the hands of the nitwits. And, as for the gray hair, there was always Grecian Formula, except I couldn't stand its taste.

I was left wondering in those days, as I am today, many years later; what happens to a normal man when he gets elevated to a high network position? Watson was a sensible, 50-ish man's man. He had a department—boxing, running smoothly and getting top critical and rating numbers. Why would he put up a series of incompetent boxing-ignorant men to harass and control me? Why? Was it good for NBC? For Watson? No, it created problems where there were no problems. And finally he turned to a truly mad-dog type of rule-by-abuse executive, Ken Schanzer, whose sole qualification for a top sports job was that he was a lobbyist in Washington for the FCC. Where is the reason in that? Watson was no dope. Surely he could see that Schanzer would not quit until he got Watson kicked out, and he would take his place.

In the end Schanzer did just that. After the Seoul Olympics, for which we won seven Emmys, Watson was fired the next day. Watson, the good guy, proved no match for a lobbyist. He went home, had a brain aneurism, and died!

CHAPTER 16

Don King:
The Mane Man

There is a common misconception in boxing that Don King and I don't like each other. This is patently not true. At least on my part, it isn't. I regard King with a kind of fatal fascination, a grudging respect, and a great appreciation for his talents. I regard him with the same respect and awe that I regard a mamba snake from the Amazon, colorful but fatal. The best way to befriend King is at a distance—a great distance.

King is in the mold of all of the great con men and promoters of the ages. (Aren't they the same thing?) In a goofy way, he is physically attractive. His smile would warm the cockles off a Gleem toothpaste ad man. King's trademark—his hair—is highly original. The American public had never seen it before. The Africans in Zaire were frankly scared by it. Children cried; horses and wild animals bolted. Its effect is that once you see Don King, you will not forget him.

In 1967, King was charged with manslaughter by the State of Ohio and put in the penitentiary after he got in a fight with a man and knocked him out cold—forever. Then, after serving his time, he was released, a free man. He stepped out of prison wiser and found himself suddenly drawn to, and qualified for, the boxing business.

King used his jail time wisely. He got his higher education by reading the collected works of William Shakespeare and the King James Bible at the expense of the taxpayers of Ohio. Somehow this qualified him to be a boxing promoter.

Sure, King has a criminal past, but it's not nearly as lurid as his rivals make it out to be. He came up on the hard streets of Cleveland, selling numbers. It was a highly sought-after trade, lucrative, and aside from having a high mortality rate, a great way to make a living. This was before drugs made the numbers business a cottage industry in the ghetto.

The more interesting story is how King ascended the mountain and attained the maximum that any boxing promoter ever attained: an invitation to the White House and a presidential pardon.

Jimmy Ellis was making an attempt to come back into the heavy-weight title picture, and he signed to fight Ernie Shavers in Madison Square Garden. Shavers was known to change managers from time to time, so it was not surprising to learn that he had been taken over by a guy named Don King from Cleveland. The rumor was that King was connected, but that does not disqualify you from anything in the business of boxing. I was prepared to meet yet another numbers man from Cleveland, but I was totally unprepared for what I saw.

I met King on a sidewalk in New York, outside the Garden, walking with his fighter. At first I was struck by his imposing height, well over six feet, four inches, and, of course, his stand-up hair. The most impressive thing about him, however, was his suit. It was made out of an iridescent orange, which changed colors as he walked by the well-lit storefronts. First it was red, then a pinkish orange, then fuchsia, then vermilion red, then a ghastly puce color. As an artist, I was drawn to the suit as I was drawn to Kokoschka Expressionist painting. I have never seen anything like it anywhere.

This garish man, looking like a used car salesman, turned out to be one of the sharpest negotiators I ever met. And he had laid a trap for Angelo Dundee's fighter. We stepped into the ring for an easy win and ended up with a hard first-round knockout. Ellis was stretched out on the canvas, and King was on his way.

Time passed. Foreman was the champion; Ali was the contender. The money was monstrous for the time—$5 million for each fighter—and the promotional possibilities boggled the mind. Having been bitten by the Hollywood and New York sharpies on the first Ali–Frazier mega fight, Herbert Muhammad and the Muslims decided that they would manage the money part. Somewhere, somehow King emerged from the fog. He has never been as brilliant as when he thought up the idea of an all-black promotion. It hit the right note. A black champion, a black contender, a black country to fund it—Zaire—what was left? Voilà! A black promoter to promote it.

It was the best work I've ever seen King do, and I've watched him pull off some miracles. The folly in Zaire has been well documented elsewhere. Things didn't turn out anything like they should have. The main thing that turned out wrong (for the bettors) was that Ali upset Foreman, a five-to-one favorite, and was crowned king of the heavyweights. And Ali took with him his newest discovery—a black promoter.

Frankly, we all cheered. Finally, we thought, boxing can have a fresh start. Blacks dominate boxing in the ring, but blacks have never handled the money. It was, as King says in one of his more enlightened racist monologues, the plantation days perpetuated into infinity. The black man works the fields; the white man sits on the veranda with his mint julep, counting the cash. He wasn't wrong. It was time for the black man to administer the cash and for the boxer to get a fair shake.

Oh brother, there is nothing so misplaced as optimism in boxing. We all thought we had turned over a new leaf! What suckers! It was a new leaf in an old book.

King didn't take long to apply the rules of math he learned running numbers in Cleveland to the rules of ring economics. He was amazed to find that they were almost indistinguishable. Given his impressive size, his dynamic personality, his drive, his ambition, and his unashamed use of racism, King threatened to take over boxing in a few short years. All he had to do was stay on the good side of Herbert, Muhammad, the Muslims, and Ali. It seemed an easy thing to do.

They had not begun to cut the money pie that was Ali when snags developed. Again, faulty mathematics was an issue. Another issue was that the promoter couldn't have an ego bigger than the star. The star in this case was Ali, and nobody was bigger than Ali. Some questionable scams came to light; the take was a tad light at times and always tardy. One thing led to another, and before long Ali went back to Arum, or to anyone who would come up with the money, because the truth was, King needed Ali, and Ali needed no one.

No sooner had Ali faded from view than King found another gold nugget, perhaps not as bright, but certainly more profitable in the long run. He discovered Larry Holmes. Holmes was a shy former sparring partner of Ali's from Easton, Pennsylvania. He was huge and had a beauty of a jab, a strong chin, and the heart of a lion. He was borderline innocent, and because he had been with the Ali circus through our travels, he had come to the attention of King.

A marriage was made between King and Holmes. As in all unhappy marriages, the stories vary depending on whom you listen to, but it is generally conceded that both parties had a rare love-hate relationship going. Part of Holmes's fascination with King was his ability to command high figures, his ruthless negotiations, and deep down, inside the lion heart of Holmes, a real respect—if not fear—of King, the street fighter. It was one thing to face eight-ounce Everlast gloves, and another to face a snub-nose .38.

Let me hasten to add that many fighters have enormous respect for King because of his record and his tough-guy history, but I believe it's been years since King actually had to use force to get his way. He has a first-rate mind. He doesn't need a gun, although from time to time, he needs a bodyguard.

King's power with boxers comes from who he is, what his record is, and, more importantly, what he represents right now. And for those of you who have not followed his interesting career, what he represents to a ghetto kid is *power*, pure and simple.

King's hold on the white elite is more mystifying because they should know better, but they don't. King plays the skin game better than any man I have ever met, North or South. If it's an argument with a black man, he can invoke the specter of the white man and beat him to death with it. If he is not getting his way with a white man, he becomes the poor black being taken advantage of by the master race white man. Any angle you want to take, King has thought of, and improved upon it.

✗✗✗✗✗✗

Do you want to know how sharp and clever King was? About the time that I was given the job of boxing consultant with NBC, the McDuffie riots had broken out in the Overtown District of Miami, where my office was. In the ensuing conflagration, my little ghetto office was burned to the ground.

For the purpose of building a better facility, before the fire I had bought a double lot across the street from my office. It was worth about $50,000, and the object was to phase out my practice by moving it into this building.

After the fire I decided I had had enough. I wanted to donate this property to whomever would build a medical facility there. I wanted a black doctor to staff it with black nurses and technicians. I offered to work there at no salary until the new man was broken in.

I made the offer to the city of Miami, the Governor of Florida, and Muhammad Ali and Herbert Muhammad. I received no answer from anyone. King offered to put up the $100,000.

If you have followed the story to this point you can see why I couldn't accept it, in spite of the fact that NBC chief Arthur Watson magnanimously allowed me to accept it, knowing it would not color my negotiations with King in the future. But I couldn't take the money, because it would be dishonest of me to take it even with the understanding that it would, in no way, obligate me to King. Even if I said that, wrote it, and published it, King would still think he had an edge.

The reality is that King would have never made the offer if I weren't buying fights for NBC. That's really all you have to know.

✗✗✗✗✗✗

I've had my fights with King, I've had my good times with him, too, and I still find him a fascinating man. If he had headed for Hollywood when he got out of the joint, instead of to New York, he would probably be the head of a movie studio by now. If he wanted to, he could be successful at a variety of things, but apparently he was like all of us, bitten by the bug of pugilism. The bottom line is King is an unusual personality and, love him or hate him, you have to admit the man is bigger than life. At least, his hair is.

CHAPTER 17

Korean Fiasco

The year 1988 arrived with great expectations for NBC Sports. This was to be our defining moment. This was to be for Watson and Weisman what the previous Olympics had been for Roone Arledge and ABC: a major hit.

Originally Ohlmeyer had been signed away from Arledge and ABC to bring his magic to our NBC coverage from Moscow. However, a certain unpleasantness in Afghanistan made President Jimmy Carter pull us out of the Olympics. I had come aboard when Ohlmeyer was putting together a broadcast team of new faces at NBC. Now I was in a superb position to capitalize on the 1988 Olympics. Albert and I had bonded into a wonderful team; Weisman, my pal, was one of the top bosses; and David Neal, a big upcoming talent and a comrade, was heading boxing. What a great moment for us.

For the boxing venue, historically a hot spot of action, Weisman went out and hired a jewel. The roughest, toughest newsman in New York was unquestionably the argumentative, feisty Wally Matthews of *Newsweek*. As Lyndon Johnson said, "Better to have him inside the tent pissing out, than outside pissing in."

Wally was a youngish 30-year-old and very handsome, and built like a linebacker with a linebacker's mean disposition. He was snarling and disbelieving. He challenged everything he was told. He dug deep.

I was so sure this was going to be the highlight of my television career that I decided to keep a day-to-day journal. In light of the disaster we experienced I decided to put it in a drawer and forget the entire painful experience.

Now, looking over my last 25 years, I find I can capsule some of the hard moments and look at the cartoons that almost cost me my life.

Goodbye, Mike I. Cohen

About a week into the games, I was in our trailer when I got a call from Monaghan that blew the tempest right out of the teapot.

"I hope you're sitting down," said Monaghan, a man not to joke around when things got tough. "Got a call from New York just now, and our friend Mike Cohen just died of a heart attack."

For once I was struck dumb. A sledgehammer hit me in the forehead. I couldn't talk. Monaghan kept going.

"He went to one of those softball games he was always organizing, and he tried to stretch a single into a triple. He keeled over at third base and never made it back. I felt you had to know. I haven't told Weisman and Marv yet."

Neal popped his head into the truck.

"Jay is here ready to run through a few fights with you—"

He stopped as he saw my face.

"I can't go. Mike Cohen just passed away. I need an hour or so…"

Neal nodded and left, sensing that I needed to be left alone with my thoughts.

After calling my wife, Luisita, to see if anything could be done for his widow, Linda, I sat, locked in thoughts of Cohen, the seemingly indestructible bear of a man. Just three days before, Luisita told me that a publisher had called to have me send a copy of the movie script I had done called *The Comeback*. Cohen had insisted that he see it for book possibilities. Cohen continued to try to help me out in my various projects out of friendship but never for monetary gain.

To make it worse, all of his NBC friends were in Seoul, Korea, and not available to help his widow and children. If we had been home, they would have needed an auditorium to hold Cohen's funeral.

It did not help my regard for TV people as decent people when I approached one of the top guys and suggested we organize a top-dollar affair for Cohen's widow when we got back to New York. I got back a logical, if heartless, answer, "By the time we get back, three or four dinners will have been given and it won't mean anything. The time will be past." Bullshit. The time is never past for a little extra cash for a widow.

Well, the average age of the young lions at NBC was in the 30s, and they were reveling in their newfound success and fame, most of which Cohen got them. Maybe they thought the high, hard fastball was the way to look at life, but, sadly, they were wrong.

We all owed Cohen a great deal. Plus, the timing is never wrong to show what he meant to NBC. And a few thousand bucks can always come in handy when the widow has three small children to bring up. It comes down to the fact that one cannot put off responsibilities; one should always pay one's bills. We all owed Cohen a mighty big tab.

If We Make It Out of Here Alive...

I will not review the screwing we got at the hands of jingoistic Korean judges, referees, and Korean Olympic authorities.

However, one stands out because of the bizarre finish. A Korean bantamweight, Byun Jong-II, in a foul-filled, wrongly refereed bout, lost a decision to Bulgarian Alex Hristov.

The Korean officials and security forces physically attacked the New Zealand referee, Keith Walker, who barely escaped serious physical injury by diving for a homebound plane.

And just how did Byun Jong-II take it?

Sitting down, that's how. Sitting quietly in a corner, on the canvas, head bowed as the bizarre scene of the Walker beating ensued. He spoke to no one. He sat stoically amidst hysterics. He expressed himself in a nonviolent way that would have made Gandhi proud.

Unfortunately, as this dragged on to abnormal lengths and the immediate danger was past, we started reaching for gallows humor on our broadcast. Some skilled researcher found out that the Olympic record for sit-ins is 54 minutes. (Where do they find these researchers?)

From time to time, as we covered the bizarre unfolding events, we cut to Byun with a superimposed time clock. Almost an hour passed.

"OK, guys," said the weary voice of Neal in our ear, "time for the wrap up sitting at our positions."

The crowd was still in their seats, unreasonably expecting some satisfactory resolution to what they perceived as the greatest screwing in Far Eastern history since the Boxer Rebellion. They wanted Walker to be brought back in chains and beheaded, perhaps. Nothing less would do.

Meanwhile in the ring, Byun just sat in the same position, with the clock ticking on the screen quickly approaching world-record sit-in time.

"I'm expecting the movers to be here in a moment to cart him off," I said, editing my thoughts as I spoke.

Suddenly, the lights in the gym went out. Total blackness. The only lights were our television lights. The moment is frozen in my mind. Albert and I looked at each other. We were uncharacteristically silent. I was praying.

"You guys want to come in?" asked the concerned voice of Neal. "You don't have to stay there."

Meanwhile, I heard the feed from Control Central. It was Weisman, talking to Neal.

"Are you nuts? Tell him to talk. Wrap the show. It's great television; it's Emmy time."

"It's murder," I said.

"That too," said the compassionate Weisman. "Hopefully." (Mike didn't get to be an executive producer of NBC at 35 being a softie.)

Albert cleared his throat, straightened his tie, looked thoughtfully into the camera, and said: "This being the last will and testament of Marvin Albert, I do bequeath my entire tape library of Knicks games to my son, Kenny—"

"Get serious," Weisman, now on top of the event, said in our headsets.

We stumbled on, trying to recap the bizarre events of the past hour, behind us the stoical presence of Byun still in the ring, by this time he has definitely broken the all-time Olympic sit-in record. Someone got him a chair. He continued to sit, although now, it didn't somehow seem as serious or as official. A sit-in in a chair? Come on.

All of the cartoons I drew I offered to Monaghan, the head of NBC Sports Press. He put them up on the bulletin board to give the hard-working press a laugh. He sent them back to New York, where the local papers printed them.

In an unprecedented move, someone from the Korean press made copies of the cartoons and printed them in the Korean paper. They seem to exemplify the "Ugly American" attitude to the outrages we had just witnessed at Chamshil. Far from being apologetic, the Korean press was pissed.

By the next day, the Korean press had tracked the fact that NBC had shown the debacle on five different segments, including on Bryant Gumble's *Prime Time* on succeeding nights.

"Enough is enough," cried one Korean newspaper. Why is the American press pounding this to death? It is a national disgrace, and it is being blown out of proportion.

"It is the way we do things," said a hapless Monaghan, sent out to face a hostile Korean press alone. "NBC has attempted to present balanced coverage of Korea and live Olympic games."

Monaghan stood unflinching, facing the crowd, waiting for his inning to arrive. After a few minutes, it did.

"Why is it that all Americans hate Koreans? Why does NBC particularly hate Koreans?"

The crowd of reporters was surging forward, getting testy.

"I'm out of here," said Monaghan, exhibiting a good Irish sense of survival and fled the scene.

Meanwhile, all week the issue simmered. One Korean newspaper actually printed a full-page editorial dissecting and analyzing the referee's table cartoon. I was borderline embarrassed, but professionally happy. Any cartoon that sees print is a good cartoon in my book and good for the ego of a professional cartoonist.

The Great Robbery

Roy Jones, the American light-middleweight, was scheduled to fight against Korea's Park Si-Hun. The arena was packed with orderly Korean fans and boisterous American fans (mostly GIs). The Koreans had apparently been told to behave. They are by instinct a kind and courteous people, and their rude behavior of the past days was due to an incendiary situation in their press and television, which had overreacted to American press coverage of the disasters of the Chamshil Gymnasium. As stated, their ire seemed to be focused on NBC in general, and Wally Matthews and me in particular.

On Saturday night before the finals of Sunday, we experienced a rare thing. A night off. The first in many weeks of continuous combat. We were invited to join the NBC hoi polloi and mix with the swells who footed the bills. Translation: Dinner with the NBC executives and the advertisers.

I was seated at a front table with Watson, the cheerful, unflappable Irish politician we were fortunate to have as our leader, and with

Weisman and Terry Ewert, the producing team, which was struggling to give us creative originality and beauty and succeeding. I was irretrievably enmeshed in a ghastly no-win conversation with a sponsor's wife over the fatuousness of plastic surgery for the middle-aged man, when I was tapped on the shoulder by a security person and asked to step outside. Relieved and happy to extricate myself from a losing battle, I went with him to the hallway where I ran into the captain of our killer security team.

He was a huge man, a handsome cross between Sebastian Cabot and Larry Csonka. He had been undercover most of his life and had the scars to prove it. I will say this, when NBC went out to get the best to protect us, they got the best.

Here was the story. American boxer Todd Foster had befriended a Korean student, and they had become brothers. On this night, the student had come to the boxer's dorms and sought out Foster. He asked him not to go to the Chamshil Gym the next night because a serious do-or-die attempt was going to be made by the students to shoot Matthews and The Fight Doctor. Kenny Weldon, Foster's trainer, heard about it and called. Matthews took the call for me.

The big man had his operators around him, and they seemed in control of the situation. I was not as sure. Being the target brings up questions that do not occur to the people who are not the immediate bull's-eye.

We discussed the pros and cons, and it boiled down to don't worry.

Neal was called and was asked if we could get out of there as soon as the last bout was fought. Neal furrowed his young brow. Producers think in terms of television needs, not human life.

"Well, we have to do the close… the wrap for Costas… the other close for Bryant, and then the wrap show…"

So much for human life.

"Listen," said the giant, "I'd feel very bad if something happened to you. I've never lost a man yet, and I'd hate to start now."

"Me too," I said, resigned to my fate.

Matthews, the tough New York street kid, smirked.

"They'll never lay a glove on us, Doc."

That's why they pick young men to fly missions. I passed on dessert and headed back to the Chosin Westin, full of apprehension. Did I really need this kind of shit? I'd survived the riots of pro boxing, the deadlier Miami Overtown Riots. Why should I come to an innocuous thing like the Olympics and have to worry about my immediate health?

"Does this remind you of the Ali circus days?" Albert asked in the opening.

"Not until now it didn't," I answered truthfully.

Death threats are something anyone who traveled in the halcyon days of the Ali circus can relate to.

The Roy Jones fight was a blowout. Jones won the gold medal, hands down. Or so we thought.

And then it was over. The final bell for round three sounded, and Jones leaped into the air in triumph with his arms up in the traditional victory exultation. The coaches were equally ecstatic. Another gold medal seemed safely tucked away.

The black side of my Iberian soul took over.

Yes, Jones certainly looked like a sure winner. Yes, it should have been a sure winner. But—

I looked across the ring into the eyes of the American ref-judge Elmo Adolph. He looked pissed. He gave me a shrug and a shake of the head.

"If Roy Jones has not won this fight, then there is something rotten in Korea!" I said, going on record *before* the decision.

The Korean fighter and coaches were congratulating Jones on his masterful performance. The crowd was politely, courteously subdued.

The last round Jones had battered Park 36-14. It was in the words of Pat Putnam, "a serious whipping." That it was.

Then came the scoring:

Gvadjava was impressed, he scored it 20-18, a two-point round. Jones.

Pajar had it 20-19, a one-point third round. Jones.

That was good news.

Now Jetchev's boys lying in ambush closed the trap.

All three had Park, the befuddled Korea, winning the third round by one point!

There was a momentary hush when the ref lifted Park's hand—like a collective sucking in of air by the assembled and shocked spectators. Even the referee seemed surprised and embarrassed. The stunned Jones put his face in his hands and cried. Coaches Adams and Ken Johnson jumped into the ring in protest. Even the Korean fighter and his coaches seemed embarrassed. At the medal ceremonies Park took his medal, held it up with one hand, pointed to it, and then to the somber Jones.

"This belongs to you," he signaled. Jones could not muster a faint smile.

"This is the greatest robbery since Brinks and the Great Train Robbery combined," I said to the TV audience. For once my sense of exaggeration fell short of what I wanted to say. I wanted to cuss. Good ol' street, ghetto cussing was called for. What a jobbing!

A Close Call

Years later, when the 1988 Olympics were a dim memory, I had an early morning flight out of Miami and found myself with time to kill, having a Cuban expresso at La Carreta Café in the concourse.

A large, heavyset man in a trench coat came up to me, "Hiya, Doc. Remember me? I was in charge of your safety at the Seoul Olympics. You know we had four serious attempts on your life. Three we nipped in the bud, but that fourth guy was a kamikaze, and he almost got you that night."

Oh really? Foster's Korean pal had warned us. Matthews and I were the targets. Matthews was free to roam around, a moving target, but I was stuck in one position. I was a fixed target.

We got through the night without gunfire, and the auditorium had emptied out. Somewhere, out there in the darkened seats was a young Korean kamikaze punk with a loaded gun. Albert and I were stuck at ringside.

The huge auditorium was dark and silent. We stood in our broadcast positions in the glare of a spotlight. It was decidedly stupid to stand there. Our young producer, filled with his mission to have us do a good-bye finish, had us stand there. Awful minutes ticked by. The finish was bullshit. It could have been shot by our trucks in full safety, yet the nearsightedness that affects young mindless producers to get the shot kept us waiting. Another thing, we were on tape, so *anytime* we did it was OK. Somehow we did it then and escaped unharmed, no thanks to the shortsightedness of an unthinking producer.

"You don't want to know how close that was," said my protector. A close call, for nothing.

We rode home convinced that we had done an Emmy-award winning job in boxing. I was disgruntled because as the Olympics wore on, Albert got closer and closer to Neal, who was young and impressionable, and I began disappearing from the telecast.

Soon, every debate went Albert's way, and in the back of my mind, I saw the writing on the wall. The executives who didn't want boxing were winning. Boxing was being phased out.

Then the men in charge of boxing started being replaced. Watson was out, and Dick Ebersol, the man who invented and made *Saturday Night Live* a big hit, was moved in to take Watson's spot. He called in Weisman and said, "I got to put Terry O'Neil in your place. Terry is a good friend of my wife, and he was in the room when our child was born."

Stunned, Weisman blurted out, "If I had known that *obstetrics* were part of the job profile I'd have gone to medical school."

That was pretty much it. I knew the glory days of boxing were over. As network TV shrunk away from boxing, cable TV picked it up and saw its saleable potential. HBO, ESPN, and Showtime began to feature boxing. It was a smashing success. The networks had made another programming boner.

CHAPTER 18

From NBC
to St. Tropez

In 1989, I was called to O'Neil's office for a chat. I knew he did not like my style of openness, the freedom to say what I believed, which I had enjoyed under Ohlmeyer and Weisman, and my unique way of reporting a fight, in which I seek a storyline, orchestrate a plot, and make an adventure out of two young men who come to seek fame and fortune on NBC-TV. A fight to me is a *story.* It is very basic.

He was slight, youngish, Ivy Leagueish, bespectacled, and very earnest. He really needed a pipe to punctuate his speech with in order to convey the proper professional tone.

"What I'd like to see is a bit of a change, more toward the technical side of boxing."

"Technical side? Where is that? Technical? You hit someone; they hit you back."

"You know. Like how many inches away should you be when you throw a jab? How far, by measurement, must it go to gather force and be effective? You know, Doc, measurements. The public loves detail."

As if O'Neil had even seen a boxing match! I closed my eyes. What was the point of arguing with this guy? Another nascent network nitwit. What difference did it make, because I was toast, no matter if I took a yardstick into the ring with me. Pure nonsense.

"Terry, boxing is not tennis. We have no boundary lines, no figures to guide us. Boxing is very basic. The combatants are trying to *hurt* one another, to inflict physical damage. It's a *fight,* Terry. Have you ever been in a fight? There's no time for measurements. There are no measurements. You throw a punch from anywhere you can and land it with as much force as you can muster. The object, again, Terry, is to win the fight by hurting your opponent more than he hurts you."

I felt like I had to say something to the lad. He was trying to be an executive producer. He wanted a dialogue with me. You know, before you fire a guy.

"Well, you know what I mean. I want something more technical," he blurted out doggedly. What difference did it make what the answer was.

"Gotcha, Terry," I said, a vague promise in the air that I would mend my errant ways and do something stupid to satisfy the ill-defined yearnings of a man fully ignorant of the sport of boxing, because, ahem, he was the *boss*.

Almost coincidentally with the new crossroad came an offer from an unthought-of area: cable TV. If network TV was the past, cable TV was the future.

Boxing had taken a right turn. Networks had small budgets, and the fights were in the $50,000 to $100,000 range by now. No *good* name fights existed for that chickenfeed. Certainly *no* little fights existed for that small a figure.

It's always been my contention that if you wake a network nitwit in the middle of the night and yell, "Boxing!" at him he responds automatically yelling, "Heavyweights! Well, no self-respecting heavyweight would fight on network TV for $100,000. Forget meaningful heavyweight fights and dispel the notion of a title fight.

Networks made a choice to phase out boxing because they had to. It no longer made economic sense. Sponsorships were down, ratings were down, and revenue was down. Conclusion: bye-bye boxing on network TV, and good riddance.

Cable TV did not need sponsorships. Cable TV needed people in their homes to buy subscriptions. To what? Old movies? No, cable TV was tailor-made for showing sports. The basic blue-collar worker stays at home and watches sports on TV. Bingo! Boxing became the bait to lure people in to watch cable.

✗✗✗✗✗✗✗

Remember Barry Frank? He called to say Showtime wanted me to help him do an Evander Holyfield fight from St. Tropez. The money was good, and we'd be in the hands of Jim Spence, the ex-ABC president of sports, with David Dyles and Jim Lampley as the broadcast team. Frank felt it was a shot in the dark, but, because he believed, as I did, that my days at NBC were numbered, I acquiesced.

I never questioned wisdom from Frank. I liked the idea of helping out a new cable TV company, bringing them credibility and helping to establish a right way to do fights. And, beside that, it was summer and I had not been to Europe for my annual frolic, and I found I could take Luisita and Tina. All in all, it was one of the best moves I made in my career.

✗✗✗✗✗✗

My first meeting with Showtime was very nice and cordial, and I instinctively liked all of the brass, particularly the boss, a young lad named Jay Larkin. He had a cordial, decent, nice-guy way about him, and he looked like he was green to the ways of big-time TV, by which I mean he was not yet on the path to being a network nitwit. My evaluation of him was correct. He was a great guy to work for 10 years before he assumed the mantle of greatness and became a 100-percent network nitwit. I'll settle for those figures. Ten years is a long, long time to be a great boss in any business, especially sports TV, particularly boxing.

Larkin was basically a song-and-dance man. Small, but attractively normal, he aspired to a life in show business. He had been in Broadway musicals in minor roles. He performed at the Playboy Club in New York and then took over booking the entertainment at the clubs. On a whim, he went to Showtime for a job.

This, as you can see, immediately gave him the credentials and the credibility to take over as the head of Showtime Boxing. Such is life in the fast lanes. Anyhow, my gut feeling was very good about this kid. He looked like he wanted to learn, did not act as if he knew it all, and had surrounded himself with top boxing talent, so he fit nicely with what I would do at his age if providence had dropped me in his place.

✗✗✗✗✗✗

We had what passed for a production meeting with everyone introducing themselves and a bit of a pep talk by producer Jim Spence. It was a uniform boxing card in that all of the fights sucked. A name fighter against a nobody. A typical fight card made by network executives, not people with boxing know-how.

I had told Larkin that I worked without censorship or restraints, and I said exactly what I thought.

"Well, sure, that's why we hired you," he said blinking and shrugging. I felt better already.

"Another thing, I won't call or have anything to do with a George Foreman fight."

His face dropped as if I had tap-danced on the flag.

"Why?" he managed to choke out.

"He's a fraud. His fights are rigged or out-and-out fixed. They'll get him KO-ing these frauds. You got him fighting on Showtime, and you will have the public and yourselves believe he is genuine and that will get him a championship shot, a legitimate title fight."

"What's wrong with that?" Larkin was already starting to think like a network nitwit. How little it takes.

"I'm on a boxing safety crusade at NBC. I have accomplished much. Because of my experience with Ali and others, I have seen many a great fighter fight past his time and get seriously hurt. Or they retire and then five years later want to come back. This is when the damage to the brain is big. So I've got many boxing bodies saying you can't box beyond 37 years of age. Can't retire and then come back after two years in retirement.

"George Foreman is way beyond 37, and he has been out of boxing for 10 years. But because he was a heavyweight and famous, everyone has dropped the rules and now the gates are open once again, and old beaten-up ex-champions are stumbling out of the barn ready to take real beatings. George Foreman is slime in my book."

"Oh, sorry I asked," said Larkin, and I had the feeling that all of that went over his head. Boxing safety was not his priority; ratings were! Welcome to boxing on TV.

We were invited to dinner with Spence. We found a nice little sidewalk café on the harbor side and settled in to have a nice, controversy-free dinner. No sooner were we past our cocktails than Spence fixed me with his "I am your superior" stare.

"You know, Doc, I am one of your biggest fans," he said. "I picked you over Gil Clancy and a bunch of others because of your background, with Ali and all, and your fine work with NBC for the past decade." He paused and I waited for the "but" that precedes bad news. Spence's smile was fixed. "*But*—I must say I disagree violently with your holding two jobs at NBC. One, you make the fights as their boxing adviser, and then two, you call the fight on TV. Now, that is blatant conflict of interest and unethical."

There was a pause in the conversation as we ordered our meal. His wife charmingly chit-chatted with Luisita, who knew a storm was brewing in my head. I smiled the same phony TV smile at Spence.

"I quite agree with you. It was a conflict of interest, yet in 10 years no one caught me putting on a bad fight and calling it good. Now, I will freely admit to you that it was unethical if you will admit what you and Roone Arledge did when called to testify about rigged and fixed Don King fights was blatantly illegal. Lying under oath to Congress carries five years in jail. You didn't go to jail for lying, did you?"

Spence turned a few shades of red. He knew I knew what that balls-up scandal was all about, and because the press did not choose to run with it, it was laying there like a ticking time bomb. What was the point? All of the media knew King was crooked. So what if ABC didn't?

Years earlier, according to informed sources, King had made a contract with ABC to produce a tournament aboard an aircraft carrier. The idea was good, but no one counted on the slipshod crooked way that King picked the fighters. He altered records. He changed names. He put in ringers, he out-and-out fixed the fights so the results would produce a more attractive series of bouts. King at this time had not yet purged himself of his criminal mindset, and he saw nothing wrong in a little fudging. I'll say right here that King would never stoop to doing that now. He is the best promoter in the world and doesn't *need* to. But then, he was fighting for his life as a promoter, and he desperately needed to have a successful tournament for ABC. Ergo, a little King trickeration.

What followed has widely been claimed and disclaimed. I am not a court of law. I can tell you what the prevailing wise-guy opinion of what happened was, and what the result was, and you draw your own conclusions. No one went to jail.

ABC had hired a gold mine in a brilliant young intellectual, Alex Wallau, who had gotten a fine education, but he had a penchant for vulgarity and was drawn to television, worse than that, *boxing* on television.

Wallau, using his contacts and suspecting the worst, dug deep and came up with all of the horrible facts, and being a good company man on the rise, he put it in the hands of Spence and Arledge in the form of a white paper, dated precisely. Wallau, no dope, kept a copy.

Here is where the cheese gets binding. They read it and put it in a safe. The tournament was in mid-course and getting respectable ratings, so they decided to ride out the storm and finish the tournament. They knew it was crooked, but they chose to ignore it.

Their luck did not last. Writers popped the story, and everyone ran for cover. Except for Wallau, who had written his white paper and dated it. He had his in a safe, too.

Spence and Arledge had to appear before Congress and lie through their teeth that they never knew about King's trickeration. Of course, Wallau's white paper indicated without a doubt that they were aware of the full extent of the crookedness weeks before and continued to present King's crooked tournament.

Without even a weak denial, Spence shut up at dinner when I mentioned that. We ate the meal in strained silence and skipped dessert.

Let me state very clearly right here that I've just written was revealed to me by a very fine New York boxing writer, Jerry Lisker, the sports editor of the *New York Post*. It was accepted by the media as the truth. I cannot prove it as such. But this is what I do know:

- **Jim Spence did not deny it. And soon, he left ABC.**
- **Alex Wallau went up the ABC ladder. At one point he was appointed as an ABC boxing broadcaster, a post for which he was singularly ill suited, having had no experience at all in boxing or in broadcasting.**

Wallau had the bad luck of getting cancer of the tongue, which is a most horrible form of cancer because it requires the disfiguring surgery of the side of the face and throat. Then the prognosis was grim, at best one to two years.

I am happy to say that Wallau is still with us some 20 years later and is now the president of ABC. Do you believe in miracles? I do.

Well, that is what I was told and saw happen. Eventually Spence left ABC, and Wallau is the president at ABC. That white paper has long since been shredded. It is a reminder of a bad time in televised boxing, where network nitwits were putting their full trust in ex-convicts such as King and expecting them to act like angels. Leopards don't change their spots, and a crook is still a crook.

CHAPTER 19

Amateur Hour in Dixie

Showtime called again. I wasn't surprised, and I wasn't overjoyed. I just didn't know if it was going to become amateur night in Dixie. And frankly, I was undergoing some self-examination.

What was it I wanted to do for the rest of my life? I was healthy as a horse. My private life was superb: married to a beautiful, talented flamenco dancer with a perfect little girl I doted on and who filled me with satisfaction and pleasure, along with my other children, Dawn, Ferdie, and Evelyn, and my granddaughter, Alexis.

Having been with Ali for 17 years I had tasted the high life of the jet set, and the colorful days of the 1960s, 1970s, and 1980s. Was there more than this? Was TV fame any brighter? No, the Ali years had satisfied any desires I harbored about being known to the public, or at least being almost famous. Not that it is what it's cracked up to be; it's nice, but in the end meaningless for a happy life.

So, once again, I sat in my little ship of life, becalmed.

"Whither goest thou?" I asked myself.

"I knowest not," I answered honestly.

"We'll see," the wise old philosopher in my brain said.

For the moment, I was phasing out NBC. They simply quit doing boxing.

✗✗✗✗✗✗✗

Economically, NBC continuing with fight coverage didn't make sense. With HBO and Showtime doing all of the big fights, for big money, there was no way to compete. I'd had a long, happy run with them, and felt nothing but gratitude for those years of happiness. Hell, they added to my being almost famous.

Working for NBC that decade, I felt as if I were part of a family. We ate together, we partied together, and we rode together in the limo. No matter who the producer was, after Weisman was kicked upstairs, the next producer, Peter Rolfe, or David Neal, took over the family, and we went on bonding. We always tried to have at least one supper together, before or after a show. It made for a comfort zone of working conditions. I think each man looked forward to doing our *NBC Cross Road Fights* as a sort of family affair party.

Making solid friendships with people such as Watson and Cohen, who are no longer with us but missed just the same. Weisman, Rolfe, Neal, Albert, and Monaghan. Today, when I write this, I'm still in touch with all of them.

When I had a stroke in 2003, 17 years after NBC dropped boxing, everyone at the network from those old days called me to see how I was and if I needed anything. Now that's family. Conversely, only one person, Gordie Hall (and he was originally from NBC), from Showtime called.

As to the new guys who took over at NBC, I only really interfaced with Ebersol, whom I found to be very bright and perceptive. The first thing he did was to recognize that he had an Ali expert on board, so he structured four two-hour specials. On all of them he gave me their star producer, David Neal. Neal and I traveled alone to Zaire and did a great two-hour special. We won an Emmy for our show on the 25th anniversary of Cassius Clay–Sonny Liston. Neal was superb, and in spite of our differences in age, we got along like brothers and worked smoothly like partners. He read my mind, and I did what he asked, trusting his judgment implicitly. Ebersol got us the Emmy. Before the academy had made no recognition of the writing we, the on-camera talent, did, but Ebersol made them see their error, and I'll always thank him for that.

✗✗✗✗✗✗✗

Before we leave NBC forever, let me leave you with a priceless moment. We were in the Fifth Street Gym, shooting Chris and Angelo Dundee, "Sell-out Moe" Fisher, Sully and Raincoat Abramovitz, and the Gym Rats, when it occurred to me that ring announcer Frank Freedman was absent. I called him up and told him to come down to be taped.

"I'm not fighting anymore," said Freedman, a delicious whimsical wit. The reference to taping meant taping the hands of the boxers to him. He was 84 at the time.

"No, I mean taping for TV," I said, going with the gag.

At the appointed hour Freedman walked in, straight as an arrow, in a spiffy three-piece suit. Neal's eyes gleamed in appreciation.

"This ought to be good," I said to Neal.

He nodded.

It was a one-on-one headshot. I faced Freedman; he faced the camera. I only needed him to say that the Cassius Clay–Sonny Liston fight was the biggest night of his announcing career. He had said that to me many times. He nodded, but he looked tense and nervous.

The first three takes he struggled badly and appeared confused and disoriented. I felt sorry for Freedman, who prided himself on his diction and large vocabulary.

"Look, Frank, I'm going to cheat a little. I'll say, 'Wasn't the Clay–Liston fight the biggest night of your life?' And all you have to say is yes. That's it."

He nodded happily. He could handle that. He rearranged his tie. The makeup girl came over and put powder on his nose. He beamed. Showbiz!

Quiet on the set! Lights! Action!

I asked my question slowly. I could see the wheels turning in his head. He lifted a finger in the air, and said, "No, Pearl Harbor was bigger!"

✗✗✗✗✗✗

With NBC no longer in the picture, Showtime called again and again. I was hired, but I did not want the security of a contract. I wanted to be free to leave if things didn't go well or if they turned network nitwits on me and tried to censor or control me. The money was good, and I would not be burdened with making the fights.

After a very successful year with Showtime, I had an informal meeting with Larkin. I really liked him because he was trying hard as hell to make Showtime work, and he had hopes of overtaking HBO and becoming number one in boxing on TV. I was drawn to his ambition to be good and tried through every means I knew how to advise and encourage him. He became like a younger brother for whom you harbor a great desire to see win.

We had an odd agreement. Upon my request I wanted no contract. I could walk away if I wanted, or conversely, they could fire me if they wanted.

Our agreed handshake was simple.

"I'll stay as long as you need me," I told him. "Or I'll go if I'm not happy."

We shook hands.

"As long as I am here, you are here," Larkin said.

That worked for almost 15 years. That must be some kind of record for television. That handshake stuff works as long as both partners remain the same. Unfortunately, here they didn't.

Our working relationship was excellent at first. We had some major differences based on the insecurity at creating a Showtime persona. I decided time would bring them around to the professionalism I was used to from my years at NBC, but that was not exactly the way things worked out.

With the different people they tried out we ended up with a pretty well-defined crew, which lasted until I left. The producer was David Dinkins. He was the privileged son of Mayor Dinkins of New York. Dinkins had personality differences with almost everyone on the crew because of a curious combination of elitism and chip-on-the-shoulder racial attitudes. Dinkins had a tendency to put himself into a ghetto mentality and to look at everything through Spike Lee glasses. Everything became fodder for the racist machine.

That pissed me off. Hell, I'd spent over 20 years in a pure black ghetto, risking my life to give free medical care to old black folks and children. Dinkins had lived in a mansion. He lived with a white woman. I had rubbed shoulders with Malcolm X, Martin Luther King, Muhammad Ali, and Jesse Jackson. Who was he to turn the slightest phrase into a racist slur? How dare he challenge me on racist lines?

Once, I said if a boxer won the fight he'd be "in the tall cotton"—an old expression of having made it in the United States.

"You can't say that. It's offensive," he stated.

"To whom?" I asked, astounded that that innocent bit of Americana could somehow be linked to racism and a racial slur.

"Tall cotton somehow evokes slavery."

"Oh, grow up," I said wearily, because no matter what he thought, I was going to say it.

But this creeping intrusion into what I was going to say smacked of censorship. They could never tell me what to say or think, but he felt he had the right to tell me how to say it. Nonsense! I wouldn't have it, but still he never backed off seeing everything through an opaque racial filter.

After a bit, when our team was set, we began to have rehearsals. Not run-throughs as in NBC where a run-through was long if it lasted 15 minutes, but a total, detailed run-through, which ran on an average of two hours. It went longer if the show had more than a couple of fights; four to six hours. And these were done the day before the fight, the day of the fight, and if anxiety ran high in the truck, right before airtime. Three rehearsals for one fight? Ridiculous!

The rehearsals were exhaustive and full, to the absolute ridiculous point where Dinkins wanted to send two groups up into the ring for my postfight interview. He actually had people stand in, and I'd interview them! Absolute amateurism. All of these were simply foolish run-throughs to satisfy the anxiety of a confidence-deprived producer.

This insanity reached its peak when we started doing big primetime championship fights. Once we were in Las Vegas outdoors, and it was cold as hell. We started in the afternoon, but then the temperature sank lower as the Vegas sun sank behind the mountains. We were endlessly going over details that involved crew matters, lighting, sound, camera positions, etc. This in effect kept the talent with nothing to do but sit and wait. Those rehearsals one time stretched to eight hours. *Eight hours!* That's a massive amount of insecurity and plain old-fashioned dumbness. Alas, it was an indication of how little sensitivity and thought for his crew Dinkins had. At NBC we ran through what we (the talent) had to do and were excused. Why should we sit through a microphone check or lines check? Nonsense, unthinking incompetence.

That night of the eight-hour rehearsal, we had a Miss America to do a minute spot. This was the lady who took Vanessa Williams's place as Miss America. She came out in a skimpy cocktail dress and stood around freezing. Finally her manager went and got a big coat and some hot tea. She did her minute perfectly. Repeated it. Did it again. They said, "Great. Wait there a minute. We may want to put that elsewhere."

The lady stood in the exact camera spot for hours. I'm not kidding—hours. Finally, I saw her, teeth chattering and looking miserable and confused. All of this abuse, for one inconsequential minute on a boxing show? I called the truck, raging about her standing in one spot for hours. Didn't Miss America have to go to the bathroom like everyone else?

I got the permission to release her. They'd simply forgotten her. Nothing intentional. She smiled a frigid smile and fled. What followed I cannot exaggerate, but believe it as gospel truth.

Not 60 seconds after Miss America stepped away from her camera spot, a huge overhead light fell on the exact spot where she had been standing. It would have crushed and killed her. Someone would have had to explain why Miss America was standing in one spot on a freezing night for hours. It was a close call.

I was wearing a thick turtleneck sweater, a wool blazer, and an overly huge Union Blue woolen overcoat from the Civil War, and I was cold as hell. Finally crew workers found a piece of tarp they could put over me. It was beyond description. Nobody can be that insensitive to a crew's needs, especially because it was not necessary. There is not an experienced producer at any of the other networks who would need an eight-hour rehearsal to put on a four-hour boxing show. We not only did it that freezing horrible Valley Forge night, but also repeated it the day of the fight. I think that rehearsal was cut to six hours.

I believe the reader should know that a fight program has no time boundary in cable TV. A fight's length cannot be calibrated. No one knows how long a fight is going to last, so time rehearsals are stupid and unrealistic. A fight could last 48 minutes until the end of 12 rounds or one minute into the first round. So what is the point of rehearsing time? This is not a Broadway play! It's boxing!

The great producers of NBC just flew by the seat of their pants, but they had talent and a feel for improvising a TV show. The crazier it was, the better. There is no way to anticipate what is going to happen in a ring. Could anyone anticipate Mike Tyson biting off a piece of Evander Holyfield's ear?

Similarly, and more disturbing, as years began to pass by, there was more on-hands editing of what was going to be said at the top of the show. Steve Albert was smart and did a great opening when left alone. More and more Larkin began to interfere, changing entire paragraphs until Albert's script looked like a Scotch tape nightmare. This slipped into a total control of what Albert said, virtually taking him out of the picture. Even the worst producer at NBC would have never have dared to try that on Marv Albert. But, sadly, Steve was not Marv.

My battles were not about what I was going to say, but about how, which invariably came from Dinkins, soaked in racial overtones. I rejected that out of hand, and we never settled on a satisfactory working arrangement. Although toward the end of 14 years, he either tired of the disagreements or grew up.

As far as boxing opinions, we had no problems at all for the first half of our tenure. Then, slowly, as Larkin metamorphed into a network nitwit, he began to believe, as they all do, that because he had seen a lot of boxing, he knew all there was to know about boxing. Eventually, he began to intrude on my call, getting in my ear while I was calling the fight. To his credit, he gave it a good try with me and eventually gave up. I mark it to the night we had a top light heavyweight fighting a virtual unknown from Washington D.C., who figured to be knocked out in the early rounds.

As often happens in boxing, the underdog was a better boxer than anyone suspected; furthermore, he had the favorite's number. Styles make fights. This one had the makings of a major upset. I spotted this by the third round and started predicting that the underdog would win. The further along the fight went, the more I was sure of it. This analysis is why they pay the big bucks. So what do I get? In my earphone comes the voice of Larkin.

"Ease up on that, Doc. You have him ahead, but here in the truck [meaning him] we have it even. Don't go out on that limb."

That made me go out even further, and I confidently predicted a one-sided win. When the decision was announced, I was vindicated! A lopsided win for the underdog. You heard it here first, folks, on Showtime!

I steamed backstage, mad as hell. It was one thing for Dinkins, his judgment clouded by racial thoughts, to argue with me, but quite another to have an actor tell me what to think about a boxing match.

We met, and I ripped into him.

"Don't ever do that again. Don't ever give me your opinion on a fight. Talk to me about the way a telecast is going. Yes, that is your job as a producer. Do not presume to tell me what I am seeing. I was totally right; you were totally wrong. In the future, fuck off."

He blinked, and I am sure I lost many points, but in Larkin's defense, I must admit, he never did that again. Later, I found out he was on the intercom to Steve Albert telling him what to say, and of course, Albert didn't have any credentials in boxing, coming as he did from the world of NBA and game shows.

As the problem of these unnecessary, interminable rehearsals escalated and my patience grew thin, I complained more and more to Larkin. These rehearsals took the life out of the telecast. There was no spark, no spontaneity, no high-wire-act thrills. All of our telecasts were numbingly stilted, dull and familiar. It wasn't a live telecast; it was a final oral exam in college.

For a while I felt I had Larkin's ear. At first, when this was all new to him, he seemed to listen to me, said the right things back to me, and did nothing to change things. I also felt that he could use my long 10 years of matchmaking for NBC to help him make the right matches and look out for the pitfalls of bad and crooked promoters. But I soon felt like he wasn't listening and that he thought I was absolutely wrong in trying to help him. He didn't need help. He never asked for it. In short, I was a presumptuous jerk to offer it. Larkin, ever the diplomat, never said, "Mind your own business; who asked you?" But his deaf ear told me all that I wanted to know. With great relief, I shut up. Matchmaking for NBC had given me high blood pressure and gray hair. Being on-camera talent was all fun and no worries.

✗✗✗✗✗✗

Soon I began to notice a marked difference in the way we did things. There was a feeling of division and alienation coming from the top. Elitism is a virus that divides and tears up any effort at teamwork. As the endless, exhausting, pointless rehearsals grew in length, the time spent together shrunk to where guys simply went to their rooms and had room service or gathered one or two at a time to have a beer. Where Weisman gathered 10 to 12 guys from the crew to have supper and talk beyond midnight, Larkin was seen at a distance in a good restaurant with Dinkins or the girl in charge of publicity or the female unit manager, and no one from the crew invited. That was when a bell finally rang in my dense head.

I had been trying to bond with Larkin for all of the reasons previously stated and had turned to him to solve the problem of these harmful, never-ending rehearsals. For once in all my years in TV I singled out one guy as being at fault, and it was, of course, Dinkins. If he didn't know what he was doing, why should I pay the price?

Things take time to register on my mind when I like a guy. It's kind of like a love affair. The girl has giant warts, but you can't see them, or better, refuse to see them.

The more all of these things piled up, the more I became aware of the obvious. Where I thought I was brought in to help Larkin on the inside, it was increasingly obvious to me that I was way outside. This was carried home to me by a small slight. We had a Thanksgiving show. I had brought Luisita, and we looked forward to a crew Thanksgiving party as we had had at NBC. No invitation was forthcoming. So I took my wife to a good Las Vegas restaurant. There sat Dinkins, his wife, and Larkin having a nice Thanksgiving dinner. It was then a dim light bulb went on in my head. These guys really do think that they are superior.

All of my complaints and objections to Larkin over Dinkins's incompetence went over Larkin's head because Dinkins *was* Larkin. By this I mean the rehearsals were as much Larkin's as Dinkins's. Larkin came from the world of theater, where rehearsals were part of the job.

Once I realized that Dinkins was in reality Larkin, I knew we were lumbered. Neither guy knew how to do it shorter or more efficiently. Each needed long, drawn-out rehearsals to settle their nerves. No matter that time after time, the unexpected events of a boxing match made shambles of their rehearsals.

Although the first half of my 14-year stay at Showtime was filled with hopes and dreams that eventually they would arrive at the obvious conclusions of how to professionally do a show, the second half saw me sadly accept the fact that things weren't going to get better because Larkin and Dinkins didn't know enough to realize that things as they were were not acceptable, and more importantly, that things could get better with a little introspection, criticism, and study.

CHAPTER 20

Showtime Follies

Having started my adventures with Showtime on such a downer disclaimer, there obviously were some good times. Otherwise, I wouldn't have spent roughly 14 years with them. We especially had some nice times when we were trying very hard to be better than HBO.

Many of those nice times were due to the black shadow of King. Showtime, like so many innocent others before them, handed over the keys to the ranch to him.

I took Larkin aside and told him: "Kiss your ass goodbye. You will do what King says or you'll be toast. So the hopes that you had to lead Showtime to the big time have arrived, and it is spelled K-i-n-g."

Although I knew very well what King would do to Showtime, I found much to my surprise that I was wrong. King brought Showtime to the big time with program after program of big-name fighters in the big-time fights. All of the good champions were with King, and he gave them to Showtime. In particular, we had the great Julio Cesar Chavez in fight after fight after fight. We had Holyfield, and better than him, we had Tyson until he imploded. What a ride!

✗✗✗✗✗✗

Tyson is an enigma. He is a troubled soul—half-man, half-child, filled with self-loathing, unable to restrain his psychotic impulses. And the worse the offenses, the more antisocial behavior he demonstrates to the public and the more the public wants to see him in the ring.

What's a man to do? Is it any wonder that Tyson is confused? On one hand they could put him back in the penitentiary for five years, or

206

if the mayhem occurs inside the ring, he can get $20 million for the same outrage. Where does this troubled soul go for help? We tried to follow his tragic journey on Showtime.

In the heady days for us at Showtime, Larkin was putting on great fights. We were being recognized as a legitimate challenger to HBO. HBO and King had a falling out. King fled into the waiting arms of Showtime.

We were in Australia when we heard. Everyone was cheering except me. I *knew* King. I was still wishing for big things for Larkin. He was doing so well, building a solid boxing program for Showtime and gaining a good reputation for himself. Now, the shadow of King fell on him. Any hope of putting on independent Larkin Showtime fights went out the window.

Because Showtime was the benefactor of King's big-name fights, we had Tyson. Actually, King had Showtime as his private TV outlet to show Tyson. The MGM Grand came on board with huge bucks. For a while there it was raining bucketfuls of money on Tyson's head. Could this felicitous turn of events last? You don't know Tyson. You don't know King.

We were scheduled to do another Tyson fight, and I decided to go and visit with him for an afternoon. I didn't want cameras or tape recorders; I just wanted to visit the lion in his den.

I arrived as Tyson was finishing a video of the movie *The Silence of the Lambs*. He motioned me to sit and watch the end of the movie. We watched as he sat riveted to the screen. Finally, it was over and he turned to me.

"The book was much better."

"You read the book?" I said, trying not to sound incredulous.

"Yeah, in the book the two FBI agents have a love affair. That's better."

And, of course, he was right.

"I didn't know you liked books."

He got up and showed me a long shelf of books, mostly novels and detective stories. I was impressed, so we talked on for an interesting half hour. Gone was the snarling animal, the street lion. In his place sat a calm, charming man, intelligently discussing book after book. Finally I asked him if he read history. For example, World War II history. He made a face.

"I hate history. It's dull. Dates, names, and all that stuff," he said, making a face.

I tap-danced for a while and launched into a story.

"Did you know the Japanese almost invaded the United States in World War II?"

"No, they did? Why didn't they?" He was hooked.

"They missed what they came after in Pearl Harbor, the oil storage tanks. Without oil, the Pacific Fleet, what was left of it after Pearl Harbor, would have been immobilized; then the Japs could come back and take Hawaii, and then the U.S. invasion.

"They came steaming across the Pacific. We didn't know where they were going. Suddenly part of the Jap fleet sheared off and went toward Alaska.

"Then we had a problem. We had only four carriers waiting to engage them. But where were they going? Alaska, and invade the U.S. through Canada, or Midway? We didn't want to split up our four carriers and lose our punch. It was a tough gamble; the war hung in the balance. What to do?" I paused. Tyson was hooked.

"Well, what happened?" He bit hard.

"History," I said. "See, history can be a mystery story. I'm not going to tell you. I'm going to send you a book on Midway, and you'll read about what happened."

I sent him a *Time-Life* series of World War II. It was filled with great photos and art. I recommended *Tora, Tora, Tora,* the film. I never heard back from him. For all Tyson knew, the Japs were still headed for Midway.

I left feeling very good about the afternoon. I had found a side of Tyson that no one knew.

So it was with great consternation that I found myself on the out list at the Tyson camp for the next fight. He sent word to Showtime, that he didn't want me to interview him. Why? I wondered. What set him off?

The reason was as simple as it was childish. I had not mentioned that Tyson was an avid reader when we did his last fight. He was upset and felt I had dissed him!

We were rocketing along on the Tyson Express, having one-round knockout fights as "Iron Mike" began to intimidate his opponents so badly that they almost fainted going up the ring stairs. It was pathetic. You'd have to go back to Sonny Liston or way back to Joe Louis to understand the power of intimidation. Meanwhile, Showtime enjoyed huge ratings.

But if you are a ring historian, you know there will be a night when the boxing gods turn against you and when all your mighty reputation crumbles before the force of bad luck. The powers that be at HBO were offered many bucks to have Tyson fight in Tokyo. Tyson-san had become a huge favorite in the Orient. Tyson's people did not want a tough fight, so they picked a fat, non-threatening, average heavyweight to get knocked out. The main qualification was that he last at least a few rounds. Buster Douglas was wallowing in the midst of a distinctly mediocre career. He was big. He'd look good going down before the mighty devastating fists of Tyson. The fight opened at 100-1, and some Vegas insiders took it off the boards, others went to 200-1. Get the picture?

Watching the fight from home, I sat, resigned to the inevitable scene of falling timber. But wait. Douglas had a stiff jab. Tyson, small as he looked next to this gigantic Douglas, was eating every jab, and he couldn't get to Douglas to punch. Huh. How long could Douglas keep the jab going? On and on it went, round after round. I sat up in my chair. Could this possibly be happening? Round six came with Douglas well ahead on points. What the hell?

By round 10, Douglas was pounding Tyson with impunity. Douglas, a huge man, could punch. No one had ever really tested Tyson's jaw.

Soon, Tyson, with arms flailing around like a drunken sailor on a pitching deck, went down. He was on all fours, groping for his mouth-piece as the referee counted 10. *Tyson was out!*

This was easily the upset of the century! A 200-1 shot upsets the Man of Iron.

There was a gigantic brouhaha, but the end result held up. Douglas had beaten Tyson. Back at MGM and Showtime, they were trying to figure out whether this was good or bad. Tyson, the one-round fighter, was getting tiresome. Tyson, the defeated fighter, had to get on track. A huge fight was in the offing. Rematch. How savory.

But sometimes, when luck turns on you it never lets up. Tyson was about to take his biggest blow.

As Tyson geared up for the fights, which would lead to regaining his title, he made a misstep. It was huge.

Tyson took a beauty contestant to bed, refused to see her home, and woke up arrested for rape. The facts were so obviously in Tyson's favor that no one took it seriously. The girl had gone to Tyson's room in the early morning hours and went to the bathroom to get ready, and here stories differ. Tyson said they had consensual sex. The girl yelled rape. Next day, the girl had a lawyer with legal papers all made out, her mother and father standing by, and subpoenas served on the shocked Tyson.

After the storm this caused had abated, Tyson was sentenced to six years in the penitentiary. He had to do three years! Somebody had to give King mouth to mouth. Not even his mighty trickeration could spring Tyson.

During Tyson's three years in jail, I decided to write to him every month to keep his spirits up. I felt sorry for him. I felt he could be helped. He could be saved. He could come back and win back his title.

For three years, every month after a Showtime fight, I'd write a long letter discussing the fights and giving him encouragement. Once, I published a new World War II novel, *Renegade Lightning* and sent it to him, along with two Ali books I had published. Silence from "Iron Mike."

Then one day, out of the blue, I got a letter from him. In the letter, dated August 23, 1993, he wrote:

Hello Doctor, I just got your letter and I was so happy to see your name. Believe it or not I always liked you as a man. I just never knew how to take you, because I am a great believer we must distrust one another, it is our only defense against being betrayed.

Well, I thought. Strange. But a breakthrough.

Then came our first meeting, a production meeting to see how he would fit in with our broadcast team. He was two hours late and surly when he did show up. He did not look at me at all, and sat, eyes averted, until we were through.

I got up and dashed for the elevator. He came in at the last moment as the doors closed.

There was an embarrassing moment of silence, and then Tyson spoke, "Thanks for writing to me, Doc. It helped a lot."

That was it. We didn't shake hands or embrace.

Tyson is a strange bird.

✗✗✗✗✗✗

Finally, "Iron Mike" did his time without incident and was released. Immediately, King entered negotiations for a Holyfield fight. A few easy tune-up fights and then a mega fight.

The Holyfield fight shaped up as a great night. Tyson had knocked out every stiff put in front of him, and he looked physically and emotionally ready to win back his crown. Holyfield was always ready.

The fight was wonderful, but from the beginning I sensed that Holyfield had the correct game plan to fight Tyson, and Tyson had no answer.

Holyfield saw that he had the advantage of size and strength. He was almost a head taller; he was heavily muscled and in his usual superb shape.

Frustrated, and at his wits end, Tyson was aware he was losing the fight, and he came at Holyfield with reckless abandon. This was what Holyfield had been waiting for. He clocked Tyson and decked him for a 10 count. Holyfield had won easily. Showtime, the MGM Grand, and King held a midnight prayer meeting.

King, who could find a silver lining in the Titanic going down, stood up and bellowed, "*Now* the rematch is worth Me'yons! Me'yons!"

And, of course, it was.

The Tyson–Holyfield Rematch

Who could have dreamed that "Iron Mike" Tyson would provide us with another one-of-a-kind memorable experience? The buildup was intense, something like the old Ali–Frazier I days. The betting was heavy. Holyfield wasn't getting any younger. Tyson had something to prove: He wanted revenge.

When the bell rang, I felt an excitement I had not felt for years. I looked over at my broadcast partners, the ex-champ Bobby Czyz and the implacable Steve Albert, and I saw my excitement reflected in their eyes. Yes, this was going to be a bitch of a fight night.

From the opening round it looked to me like this was going to be a continuation of the first fight. Holyfield was following his foolproof game plan, Tyson was being frustrated and taking a methodical beating.

Suddenly I saw Tyson's head on Holyfield's. It looked strange, as if Tyson was biting Holyfield's ear. Holyfield jumped back holding his ear. Mills Lane, the great referee, looked perplexed.

"No more of that or I'll disqualify you," he warned.

Things are very confused. Did Lane dock Tyson a point? He should have. But then he'd have to stop the round and award the point deduction so the judges could see and mark their scorecards. But Lane did not do that; he waved them on.

Almost immediately they went back into a clinch. This time Tyson looked like a dog gnawing on a bone. I saw the tip of Holyfield's ear bounce in front of me.

The brown chunk of bloody meat stopped directly in front of my eyes. It was hard to believe this was a good chunk of Holyfield's ear.

"He's bitten off a chunk of Holyfield's ear," I yelled into my mike.

Czyz and Albert stared at it, open-mouthed. They were too shocked to react for a moment, and then all three of us were babbling at the same time.

"One at a time!" the truck was yelling in our earphones. "One at a time guys!"

In the meantime the bizarre drama was playing out in the ring. Lane was trying to make order out of chaos and trying to avert a riot as both corners piled into the ring with a battle on their minds. Holyfield was in the corner holding his ear.

"He bit me! He bit my ear off! He bit me!" Holyfield kept repeating.

Poor Holyfield has had some strange nights in his career but nothing could compare with this.

✗✗✗✗✗✗

I hate to say it, but aside from the Ali circus, I was never involved in as many great fights as I was with Showtime. I came to, *gulp,* love Don King. That man can promote.

Then Showtime lost King over money and through stupidity and crass, thoughtless behavior. I'll cite one example, although there are many.

We were in Mexico City. It was Julio Cesar Chavez's birthday. He was fighting a record-breaking title fight, and coincidentally it was Don King's 100th major title fight on primetime TV. I thought it called for a little extra celebratory TV show. So did King, so did Chavez. But not Showtime.

The fight went the distance. It was a damned good fight. Chavez talked a bit afterward, not long; I translated and turned to King. I wanted to do something special for him. After all, I had been part of the team that gave him his first promotional break with the Rumble in the Jungle. Here we were in Mexico City, midnight, in front of 125,000 record-breaking fans, celebrating his 100th fight.

Room for celebration, no?

"No time for King, get him off," I heard in my earphone.

I pressed the talk button, "Are you crazy? Tell King he can't speak on so big an occasion in his life?"

"Yeah. Get him off!"

"No," I said and tried to explain to King the rude hosing he was getting for no reason at all. King exploded. He should have. I found the boss of Showtime, a wonderful guy who was very fair, and offered a solution.

"Let me tape the interview with King. Then we tell him that while we ran out of time in Mexico City, we are going to play it in its entirety when it airs in America on Thursday."

The boss agreed that it made sense and to do it.

Now why in God's name would they slam-dunk King on one of his most important nights? He was our only provider of good fights. Why insult the hand that feeds you? That's idiotic, ill-tempered, ill-conceived, loutish behavior. I did not think that King deserved this boorish behavior. It's not like he was having trouble with Showtime brass. He wasn't. He was easy to work with, and Showtime was the beneficiary of his goodwill, his vast array of boxing talent, and his worldwide connections to land interesting venues. Why slam-dunk Don King?

Answer: naked, unvarnished stupidity, and I'll add, smug, smug stupidity.

I found it offensive and unforgivable.

When King left Showtime, we felt protected because Larkin and MGM had signed Tyson to a five-fight deal for $25 million. We still had a hold on Holyfield. I was certain Larkin had crossed over into a network nitwit heaven when he confided to me that if he wanted, he could take over Holyfield and manage him. I looked at Larkin in a new light. He'd been bitten by the boxing bug. He really thought he could just dip in and manage Holyfield? Oh, brother.

By this time I could see disaster coming. We gave all of those millions to a ticking time bomb? Tyson? Were they kidding?

Boom! Tyson exploded and landed in jail for three years. Oops, a little sidestep was in order. From there on out it was chaos. Not nice to see and horrible to be a part of.

More Characters from the Ring

We took our Lou Duva connection from NBC to Showtime. Duva had a workhorse in champion Rocky Lockeridge. He was small and tough as hell. We showed him many times.

When he came to fight for the title, he drew a very tough Roger Mayweather who was favored to knock out Lockeridge. Why fighters do crazy things no one knows. For these fights Mayweather bought a pair of wraparound jet-black sunglasses. You couldn't see in, but it didn't look like he could see out too far, either. Mayweather obstinately would not take them off. He went to the publicity luncheon and the weigh-in wearing his dark glasses.

The night of the fight he wore the wrap-around jet-black sunglasses in his swaggering ring walk. Duva, always looking for an edge, went crazy and demanded that he take off the sunglasses. Mayweather refused. A riot was about to ensue. Mayweather came to middle of the ring for the introduction wearing his sunglasses and did not take them off until the bell rang to start the fight.

Then he whipped off his jet-black sunglasses and was blinded by the white ring lights. He couldn't see.

Lockeridge could, and he threw one hard right punch, which landed on the blinded Mayweather, crumbling him into a heap. Knockout in one. New champion of the world.

That's odd? Wait.

The top gufus of my 40 years, though, is easily Livingston Bramble. Bramble was a scary-looking guy who sported huge Rastafarian dreadlocks. He took two pets with him wherever he went: a boa constrictor snake that he called "Doc" and a ferocious pit bull that he called "Snake." When he arrived to contend for the title against Ray "Boom Boom" Mancini, he brought his minister witch doctor. This guy had a bowler hat on his Rastafarian dreadlocks and a large walking staff. He was called "Dr. Do."

A fight broke out in the press when they saw "Dr. Do."

Dick Young, a tough New Yorker, said "Dr. Do" was a phony and should be thrown out. Elmer Smith said he was authentic if unusual, and we have freedom of religion here in the States; he should stay.

Bramble won in the late rounds with a knockout. "Dr. Do" raised Bramble's arms in triumph.

In the dressing room, Jerry Lisker, *New York Post* boxing writer, asked a happy Bramble, "Who is this 'Dr. Do'?"

"Aw, he's a basketball coach for the gym," he said, smiling with his gold tooth beaming.

"Dr. Do" raised his derby to acknowledge himself.

✗✗✗✗✗✗✗

Duva was the most entertaining cornerman in the history of boxing. He did anything to get the edge over the other fighter. One night he reached a high that even he has not topped.

In 1996, Duva brought over Andrew Golota, a very rough, tough, aggressive Polish tree trunk. Not since "Two Ton" Galento had the world seen a more menacing, more unlikely heavyweight. Duva did his act so well that he had Golota's opponent, Riddick Bowe, the champ, in a nervous tizzy.

The fight was horribly rough. It wasn't a boxing match; It was a barroom brawl—no better than that—a back-alley war. Golota hit Bowe repeatedly below the belt and even kneed the bewildered champion. Finally, to avert a boxing death, the referee stopped the fight.

Cue Duva, the human cannonball. He had forgotten to take his cardiac medication, so his pacemaker was sputtering and kicking. When Duva launched himself like the Flying Zucchini, the pacemaker gave a gigantic kick to the ribs. Duva dropped as if he had been shot by a sniper. His son, Danny, and the entire Duva clan dove for Duva, who was having trouble breathing. He got CPR and was rushed to hospital. Word around ringside was that Duva had had a major fatal heart attack. Even in death Duva was going to upstage the colossal riot going on in the ring.

The next fight, Duva was in the corner again, agitating, hollering, and looking for the edge. God love him, there's no finer character in boxing than Duva, and on the serious side, no better friend to have on your side.

✗✗✗✗✗✗

What is there about a boxing match that makes grown, sensible men risk their lives to be part of it? The next crazy man in boxing close to Duva is "The Colonel" Bob Sheridan.

Sheridan has been calling fights since 1960 when he started calling Tuesday Night Fights on Miami Beach for Chris Dundee.

For the past 30 years he has called every King fight. His call of the Rumble in the Jungle was his masterpiece. He correctly saw Ali's plan, called Foreman's futility, and predicted his knockout before it happened. The call was brilliant.

Sheridan, like Duva, is one of nature's happy spirits. Relentlessly optimistic and funny Sheridan lives in a fairytale life. He is never close to reality; he lives in Sheridan-Land, a rare place indeed.

When I saw Sheridan a couple days before Holyfield–Tyson II, he didn't look good. He was pale and couldn't breathe. I got him to go to the hospital. Sure enough, he was having another heart attack.

Come fight night he announced to the doctor: "I'm going to call the fight. It's my job."

"Like hell you are," said the doctor.

"Like hell I'm not." Sheridan ripped his tubes off and grabbed his trousers. "And you're going with me with the oxygen and all that other stuff? Call the ambulance."

I looked over from my position, and there sat Sheridan like one gigantic happy toad, barking away his call and sparkling as ever with a tube of oxygen up his nose.

And then, with Sheridan's luck, Tyson bites off Holyfield's ear. Sheridan sat up in his chair, his voice went up, and you could hear him in Los Angeles without a mike. He was in heaven, and his doctor was right with him. It's a night I bet that doctor will never stop talking about.

"What makes us do it?" I asked Sheridan back in intensive care.

"It's our job, me boy, it's our bloody job."

And, you know, it is.

✗✗✗✗✗✗

There were many pleasant memories of Showtime, especially some in Europe. Some of those nights were magic.

One night, after a near fatality in the ring, we walked the late night London streets. Larkin, with a lot of maneuvering, had gotten us permission to go into the London Medical Laboratory and Museum. Larkin and I share a fascination for the Elephant Man. So we went in at midnight to take a good look at the Elephant Man's skeleton. It was a spooky night I won't soon forget. The Elephant Man was one fucked up human being. How he lived, I don't know.

✗✗✗✗✗✗

Of all the Showtime guys, only one would visit sights to be seen. He was a former beatnik named Jody Heaps, who had washed up on the shores of Showtime as a writer. He could easily be picked out because he looked wasted like a beatnik, ate egg-white omelets and vegetables, and wrote plays. My kinda guy. His name is out of a Charles Dickens novel, where curiously enough, he would also fit. Heaps was somewhere between Eurian Heap and Mister Micawber. He was my life raft to sanity. He was funny and lively and had wonderful insights into things. He went everywhere with me, and I came to look forward to Showtime fights so I could spend time with my relic from beatnik days. He had a rich father, and I think this was the first paying job he ever had in his life. And he was 50. Jody Heaps. My guy.

CHAPTER 21

Budd Schulberg: The Modest Icon

Among the many lucky things that happened to me as I trolled my way along behind the Ali circus train was the acquaintance of one of the literary geniuses of the 20th century, Budd Schulberg.

Having been around my share of icons and self-appointed legends (Cosell springs to mind), I was pleasantly surprised to find a modest man who gave no indication of the great man that he was. We met on a common ground, our love of boxing. He did not know me at all, except, of course as Ali's doctor, so for a while we bonded together at every Ali fight.

Schulberg was a dyed-in-the-wool boxing fan. As a boy he went with his dad, movie mogul B.P. Schulberg, to all of the fights at the Olympic Auditorium, so Schulberg had firsthand knowledge of the greats of boxing in the 1920s, 1930s, and 1940s. He kept up his interest by contributing articles and special pieces. He was smart, knew boxing inside out, and better than that, knew how to put the fight on paper. Of all of the sportswriters I've met over the past 40 years, none could touch Schulberg in excellence.

Slowly I came to the realization that this quiet, modest writer had deeply influenced my life and had indeed guided me by his three best books: *The Harder They Fall, What Makes Sammy Run,* and *On the Waterfront.* All are literary treasures, on par with any piece of writing of the 20th century, perhaps better in that through his writing talent he took the reader into the real world of big-time boxing, the sleazy cut-throat world of movies, and the head-busting world of unions.

As we grew close, Schulberg began to teach me to write. Oh, we didn't have a writing class. I had 12 years of college. I knew how to write. I'd written a lot in college and in the Air Force. What Schulberg taught me was how to observe, how to infuse myself in the characters, and how to capture the blood and juices of the time and place you are writing about.

Once he said to me, "If you cut out a news item that has a strange human interest story in it, put it away. By the end of the year you'll have enough for novels, short stories, and movies to keep you busy for life."

What was he saying? Pay attention to life. Write what you know. Fiction springs from fact. He told me to start at my first memory: I remember drawing the numbers 1933 on the bow of a ship I had drawn. He asked me to start there and recall the things that happened and are etched in my subconscious. All of it. Well, since by that time I'd been in college 12 years, in the Air Force two years, and in hospital training one, the book grew to a giant book. Lots of stories!

One day Schulberg came to spend a week with me in Miami. Why, I don't remember and cannot fathom. I put a fifth of vodka on his nightstand by the bed and took him to the Fifth Street Gym to see the boxers. Ali was not in town, but I noted the ease and familiarity with which Schulberg hung in with the boxers. They didn't know who this great writer was, only that he was one of them. Quietly they accepted him, grew familiar with him, and swapped stories. Our janitor was the great champion Beau Jack. He had been the king of the New York boxing world during the war years. He hugged Schulberg as if he were a long-lost cousin.

Once at home, Schulberg said, "Show me your book of stories."

I thought he was kidding, you know, to make me feel good. I thought he'd take them home, put on a once-over glance at some of the stuff, and pat me condescendingly on the head.

Imagine my surprise when Schulberg dragged a camp chair into my backyard, loosened his shirt to get some Florida sun, put his bottle of vodka by the chair, and began to read.

I had diligently followed his suggestions. I had hundreds of stories; I am an Ybor City storyteller. We never forget a good story, and we may trim or add, but the story stays solid. I could hear an occasional laugh from Schulberg, which sent my head reeling. It's hard to make people laugh out loud at written material much less an experienced writer like Schulberg. Hearing his laugh made me feel great!

He finished the first book in a couple of days.

"Boy, that was great. I'm up to college. Does it get better than this?" Schulberg seemed genuine in his enthusiasm.

"Well, yeah, if you like college stuff. It's kind of crazy."

"Let me see it." He took book two and went out on the lawn. I ordered a case of vodka. I didn't want to run out. In those days Schulberg could consume a fifth a day without noticeable effect. He read faster, as if he were anxious to see where all this stuff was headed. He came in, red-faced, drenched with perspiration one day. He seemed perturbed.

"Did they really throw you out of Spring Hill College with only three weeks to go before graduation?"

From the look on his face I saw he had put himself into my story.

He too had a strong father, whom he idolized and never wanted to disappoint. He understood my feelings. It wasn't so much that I let down my mentor, Father Yancey, but that I had horribly let down my father. All of those years of hard work together in that hot, dusty La Economica Pharmacy and all of the hard academic work of four years and the possibility of becoming a doctor gone out the window for a prank, a pointless prank.

Schulberg was caught up in the story.

"But you did become a doctor." He seemed to be getting ahead of the story.

"Read on, it's got quite a punch line," I said happily, knowing I had him hooked.

He read on, and when he was through he was red-eyed, which I, as a doctor, attributed more to drinking vodka and staying in the hot Florida sun than to the dramatic finish of the Spring Hill story.

"Boy, what a story. See what I mean about real life. It's better than fiction. That's a good novel idea or a long short-story, and a great movie idea." He seemed moved and genuine in his praise. "See, Ferdie, you can write. You can put your feelings on paper. You have the gift of dragging the reader in with you."

He had read my three big books of life experiences. He was very encouraging.

"Put some of those Ybor City stories in short-story form; they are not only great stories, but unusual settings. The story of the lector, the strikes, and the Spanish Civil War has never been seen before. Try it in novel form. It's harder, but you have to try. The only way to write is to write."

✗✗✗✗✗✗

Schulberg began bringing a beautiful redheaded actress to the fights with him. She was his new wife, Geraldine Brooks. They were quite a pair, and we sort of fell in together.

We continued to grow closer, and now we talked between fights, and he was accessible to discuss writing, boxing, or movies.

On an Air France daylight flight to Paris, I finished reading Doctorow's *Ragtime.* In it was a fascinating character of a black man named Cold House Walker. I started to remember Sweet Sam, a black man from my youth. The more I remembered him and the mystery of the grand piano, which he never played or explained, the more I knew I had a great Christmas Eve short story.

I wrote the short story on the Air France menu, and when I got home, I had such rave reviews from my friends and writers that I had a Christmas card made, illustrated the front, and sent it to everyone.

Of special pride and joy to me was a call from Schulberg and his wife. They had fallen in love with Sweet Sam and were sending it to special people in Hollywood. The next week I got a call from Norman Lear, who was then the most successful TV producer in the land. He was sending a first-class ticket for me to Los Angeles and a suite at the Beverly Wilshire, and moreover, had Schulberg coming as well to meet and see what we could do with Sweet Sam!

The meeting was pure Hollywood. Schulberg and Lear embraced, old friends, old admirers, with Lear treating Schulberg like Hollywood royalty, which he was. Finally, it was my turn.

Lear had a lined face with kind eyes. He looked like he was on your side. He wanted you to win. With a broad smile, he tented his fingers and looked over his glasses.

"So, what do you want to do with Sweet Sam? It's a swell story. Very moving, it's true isn't it? Better. Better. What do you want to do with it?"

Why, this floored me. This producer, the king of all he surveys, has just spent over $5,000 getting us together in his office. He is the movie maven. Schulberg was a big-time screenwriter. I, on the other hand, am—am *only* Ali's doctor.

"What do I want to do with Sweet Sam? No, Mr. Lear, what do *you* want to do with Sweet Sam?"

There followed a lot of ill-defined what-if talking. Lear wanted to do something, but what?

"Is there more? Does he finally tell you why he is in hiding? Why he has run away with a grand piano and a mute wife?"

"No, the story ends when he dies on Christmas Eve after he finally plays the piano for me. If you are talking major motion pictures, I would have to invent Sweet Sam's back story. I think he was from New Orleans, and he certainly could play jazz."

"Interesting. Are you ready to do a screenplay?"

At that time I'd never even dreamed of doing a screenplay and didn't know the first thing about constructing a screenplay.

"Budd, are you willing to write with Doc on the screenplay?"

Well, that was audacious. The very thought that Schulberg, the Oscar-winning screenwriter for *On the Waterfront,* would write a script with a doctor who had never written anything professionally was laughable. Schulberg went on about a full table of previous commitments, and I felt bad because he had been put in a bad spot. I quickly demurred, saying that probably the best thing would be if I wrote the back story as a novel, and if it were as good as the short-story, maybe Lear could make it as a Movie of the Week on TV.

Thereby started the long journey of Sweet Sam. I'd never written a novel. Read a lot, but written none. I went back and dreamed up a whopper of a back story, starting way back at the Civil War, following with a New Orleans tale that was filled with Sam's charmed life as a whorehouse pianist, who on the side was inventing a new music called jazz.

This novel was rewritten at least six times, each time getting better and each time being rejected by one and all in New York and Hollywood. It almost became a film. It was optioned by an Israeli producer for big bucks. I did a damn good film script. But the Israeli's good intentions disappeared when his funds dried up. Others tried; money in, script out, money totally out. Once I had $1 million to produce it as a Broadway musical, providing, said my oil man money guy, I got Frank Sinatra to play Sweet Sam.

Now, after 30 years of selling and reselling Sweet Sam, I have re-edited out all of the New Orleans jazz whorehouse plot and picked him up with Leona on the run, where much to Sam's chagrin, he had to learn to be a Southern Negro of the 1920s.

The novel in its new form was still being turned down. This time it was the black publishers who said they didn't want stories about old-time Negro segregationalist problems in the old South. They rejected their history and wanted cutting-edge dope-laced hip-hop black dudes. Exit Sweet Sam (again).

The Story of a Miracle

One day a horrible piece of news reached me in Miami. Schulberg called to tell me that his darling wife had been diagnosed with malignant lung cancer. She was determined to fight it, and Schulberg enlisted my aid. Steve McQueen had just gone through a long and tragic course of alternative experimental cancer treatment in Paris, Arizona. He had died a horrible death.

There was nothing that could be done for poor Geraldine. After a flurry of radiation and chemotherapy, she resigned herself to dying.

I visited her at her rustic house in Quogue, Long Island. She took me to the backyard to see her swans, swimming peacefully on the still clear waters of an inlet she had personally saved as a sanctuary for fowl. It was where she was happiest.

"Promise me you won't let me die in the hospital," she said, her beautiful eyes pleading.

This was a request that was beyond my capacity. I was not her doctor and not a New York doctor. I had no medical right to interfere, if I did, I could lose my license. But, her eyes implored me and I couldn't say no. How could I?

Almost a year went by. I didn't see her, but I spoke to her once in a while as the disease took hold and ravaged her. Whenever we talked, I encouraged her as best I could. She would listen respectfully, then end with, "Remember, you're not going to let me die in the hospital."

Schulberg called to say Geraldine was at the end of the line and in the hospital. It was a mess, just as she feared it would be. Her family, the Brookses, who were renowned for producing theatrical costumes, was feuding with Schulberg. They installed themselves in a room across from hers, while Schulberg slept in a chair next to her bed. The cancer had spread, and several specialists were called in—six in all—one for every cancerous area of her body. It was a medical nightmare.

I soon got a call from the hospital in New York. I expected it to be news that Geraldine had passed, but to my considerable shock, it was Geraldine herself. Her voice was just a hoarse whisper.

"Come and get me, you promised," she said weakly.

I closed my offices for the next day, so I could fly to New York that night and be by her bedside in the morning. I knew it was madness. In all probability, she'd be dead by the time I got there, but still—I was determined to try to keep my promise.

When I walked into her room early that Thursday morning, I barely recognized her. She was pure skin and bone, a living skeleton. She had no more beautiful red hair—radiation and chemo had taken care of that. Then I noticed she had pulled out all of her IVs and catheters and was refusing medication. She was trying mightily to die.

When she opened her beautiful eyes, the light had gone out, her soul was barely holding on, but she struggled to speak. I had to lean over and put my ear to her parched mouth.

"I knew you'd come," she managed to breathe out.

"Well, hell," I thought, "I'm already here, it's worth a try."

I got the head internist on the phone and prepared to get myself roasted, but I had to try. I couldn't just take her without permission. I could get charged with kidnapping on top of losing my medical license.

"Sir, you don't know me, but I'm Dr. Pacheco from Miami," I began tentatively.

"Oh yes, I do. You're The Fight Doctor Geraldine talks so much about. At last you've come. Thank God. The family, her husband, and the specialists have been about to drive me crazy with their squabbling."

A ray of sunshine hit the phone. I was hearing all of those good words, which translated to mean, if I moved fast, I'd get her out of the hospital legitimately.

"Yes," he told me, after I explained what I was doing. "I'll file the discharge papers before anybody can object."

"Thank you," was all I could muster as I hung up and hurried to rally the nurses and to get her ready to be whisked away in the ambulance.

The trip was a suspenseful adventure. I didn't know if Geraldine would make it to Long Island, and if she died in the ambulance, there would be hell to pay from every attorney from New York to France.

Finally we made it. Her bed was ready, with crisp fresh linen, comfy and inviting. I placed the fragile little body in the big bed. She looked like a little girl in her mommy's bed. Immediately she brightened, opening her eyes and watching the sun shining on the inlet and the beautiful white swans cruising peacefully back and forth in front of the picture window. She motioned for me to lean over.

"Can you bring me some tea? The Old English on the second shelf."

Joyful over the sound of confidence in her voice, I dashed to the kitchen, made the tea, and rushed back.

"Can I have two pieces of white toast with butter?" she asked with a weak smile.

The secretary dashed to the kitchen and came back quickly. I placed a little bell by her bed that wasn't too heavy, and she could ring if she needed anything.

Five minutes passed before she rang the bell, asking for some orange tea, this time in a bigger pot, and whole-wheat toast with strawberry jam.

"Hold on, Geraldine," I told her. "I'm a doctor, not room service."

She laughed for the first time in months, and for the first time I had a good feeling about her. I kissed her goodbye and flew back to Miami, satisfied with the day's events.

Geraldine made a startling recovery. She lived four more active years in which she made a movie and several TV specials, and appeared in *Fiddler on the Roof* at Jones Beach. She died on her way to film a dog food commercial suddenly and easily.

If Geraldine Brooks's story doesn't qualify as a miracle in your book, it does in mine. The message is clear—never lose hope and never stop trying.

Friendly Connections

Schulberg teamed up with a brilliant filmmaker, Elia Kazan, to produce *On The Waterfront.* It won many Oscars, and Hollywood forgot about Sammy Glick, and *What Makes Sammy Run.*

Kazan was contentious and quarrelsome as hell. At a party at Schulberg's house in Long Island, he cornered me and launched into a long, one-sided harangue about dishonesty in boxing. He was pretty drunk; I was dead sober. So I left him at the semi-colon. Respecting the genius that is Kazan, I walked away from him and ignored him for the rest of the day.

Flash-forward about 10 years, and my daughter Tina, a film editor, and I are invited to Schulberg's 80th birthday party in New York.

Surrounded by old movie dinosaurs, like a scene from *Sunset Boulevard,* we stood observing the eerie scene when Tina noticed a shriveled old man, sinking into the deep red velvet cushions of the sofa. He curled his finger at Tina; she, knowing who he was, responded. She came back.

"Kazan wants to see The Fight Doctor," she said, wrinkling her nose.

I went over, he motioned for me to lean in toward him, and he said in a low raspy voice, "And another thing about boxing dishonesty."

He had picked up at the same semi-colon just as he had left off 10 years ago.

I'd had enough of him and his dishonesty.

"Gauge, any man who can make a great film about Zapata and then blow his credibility by making Zapata the President of Mexico has nothing to tell me about dishonesty."

So Schulberg and I have both trundled down the road of friendship; he an icon, a legend of literature and screenwriting and me almost famous and a meddler in many things. I feel blessed that I shared so many great moments with him.

I've been after him to sit at a tape recorder and spew forth the history of movie land of the 1930s, 1940s, and 1950s. His would be the true defining book. We need his memories. We need his Hollywood.

For example, World War II was over, and Schulberg was an officer in the OSS and was called to go pick up a Nazi war criminal. He hurried down to Bavaria.

He walked up the cracking staircase in a bombed-out building and knocked on the door, which opened to reveal a legend of the Nazi era, Leni Riefenstahl, who filmed the fierce intensity of the Nuremberg rallies and the speed and cleanliness of the Berlin Olympics.

"I've been waiting for you," she said in a Dietrich voice. "How is your father?" She lowered her eyes seductively. "Do you think he might have something for me?"

So, no matter where Schulberg found himself the ghost of his father B.P., the old Hollywood days, and the glory of the silver screen followed him. Riefenstahl even wanted a job!

xxxxxxx

Budd Schulberg was generally treated like a big warm teddy bear. It took a lot to make him mad, unless he was drinking vodka, which was a nightly occurrence. I had a pacifying effect on him. In fact, I was the only one who was able to put him to bed without his cracking someone's jaw after he'd had too much to drink. Once, on Budd's yacht, I kept him from popping John Wayne over a difference of opinion on the value of a Mexican bullfighter, Carlos Arruza, over Manolete, the great Spanish bullfighter. Wayne was close to Manolete, stood 6 foot 6, and was always in fighting shape. Budd was a pudgy 5 foot 10 and in shape to last no more than five minutes of hard fighting. I got between them and Wayne cooled down because he had heard I was the best boxing doctor in the world, and he had a weakness for quality. I was Ali's doctor. That saved Budd from a king-size beating.

It was always touch-and-go as to which Buddy you would get if you met him later in the night. One night in Houston, I was going to meet him for supper after he finished doing rewrites. He hated to rewrite what he knew was well written. On top of which it was a dark and stormy night. His plane coming in was three hours late and the winds were violent. But he made it.

Standing around the bar, waiting for Budd's plane to arrive, I met a tall young Swedish skier who wrote bullfighting stories for a Swedish magazine. He was kind of a bore—very opinionated and full of himself. He did not think much of Manolete.

At around midnight, with his bottle of vodka empty, Budd got off the storm-tossed plane in a rage. I hated to tell him we were eating with a Swedish bullfighting expert. It took a half an hour to cool him down. Only the fact that the Swede considered Budd the greatest writer going calmed him somewhat. Budd was simmering but civil.

Well, you couldn't tell Budd anything about Manolete, the great master. He'd drunk too many Corona beers on the plane and his end was on the way. I'd forgotten about Budd's close friendship with Manolete.

About five minutes into the Swede's sycophantic babble, smoke started emulating from Budd's nostrils and he put his fist through the tabletop and stood up.

"You boring piece of reindeer turd! You know nothing of bullfighting; you are from the wrong country."

The poor young writer was totally deflated. I had to hold Budd back. He and I had our steaks in his suite. And I never heard from the Swede again.

For ten years I had been after him to write about early Hollywood when his father, B. P. Schulberg, was one of the kings. B. P. co-founded Paramount Pictures with Louis B. Mayer. He produced the Oscar-winner for best picture in 1927, *Wings*, and had a hot affair with Sylvia Sidney. Budd then became the boy wonder who turned out *The Harder They Fall*, *Faces in the Crowd* and *Treasure of Sierra Madre*, all masterpieces of film writing.

I shamelessly used to invite Budd to all of Ali's fights. I put him in the corner next to Angelo, Sarria, Bundine and me. He was there when Ali KO'd Liston. Then he went to Kinshasa where Ali KO's the 9-to-1 favorite champion Foreman, to win back the title, then the dramatic first Ali-Frazier fight and then the greatest title fight on record, when Frazier was a whisker away from being killed. Budd, the fan, had a ringside seat. He was in the corner. Isn't it any wonder we were close friends?

Sadly, Budd slipped away and died in August 2009. I miss him every day.

EPILOGUE

When I first came to Showtime, I had a big reputation for telling the truth and for standing up for what I believed in no matter how expedient caving in to an exec's desires were. I had an open mike at NBC, and nobody told me what to say. I said what I thought was right, and I certainly expected and received no less from the struggling little cable company.

One can seldom foresee when a long relationship is coming to an end. My desire was to finish my long run on TV when I reached 75 years of age. It sounded right to me, and it would finish 25 good years of broadcasting. And because my relationship with Showtime had always been one of the warmest co-operations, I felt we would sit down and plan for my last show and make it a memorable one. After all, who had lasted 25 years as a boxing analyst? It seemed like a win-win situation to me.

Although we never sat down and discussed my disappearing act with Larkin, the whittling down began with program changes. When Jim Gray came over from NBC to do the postfight interviews, I understood the ejection process was beginning. Actually, I didn't mind it, because Gray is a first-rate talent and a friend, and I helped him get on at NBC. I was being replaced by a *name* interviewer, but I felt Showtime was shooting itself in the foot, because of my bilingual ability. As an interviewer, I could speak English, Spanish, and Don King. Besides, boxers respected, admired, and easily opened up to me. Nevertheless, Larkin felt he made the program better by implementing the changes.

The main reason that my exit had to come was they were developing a replacement, who would gradually squeeze me out like toothpaste from a tube. My choice for that honor was Czyz. Not that Larkin had asked me, understandably, but I could see that I soon would be toast.

One day, during my NBC heyday, when we had had Saturday-Sunday back-to-back shows, I had contracted laryngitis and couldn't talk above a whisper. I had spotted Czyz in the audience and had him sit in with me to help, which put serendipity in motion once again. He was great and got us through the weekend. Now, nearly 20 years later,

Czyz was slated to be my replacement, and I was cool with that. The classy way to do this was to have a meeting with Larkin, where we would discuss a graceful, honorable exit over a period of time while waiting for Czyz to get his feet wet and come up to snuff.

That's not the way Larkin chose to do it. Instead, we entered a frosty time in our previously warm, familial relationship. Larkin avoided me at every turn, if he could, and when he was unlucky enough for me to catch him, he put up a façade and was cordial as ever, but distant.

Soon Czyz was given the teleprompter to break down the fighters' strategies. That was fine with me, too, because I felt the teleprompter was a meaningless tool. Slow motion can better show you what the analyst is saying, and you avoid amateurish, jiggly white lines.

Then we were sharing commentary on what was being said in the corners, and soon, Larkin cut me out of that and left Czyz solo. By that time I felt like I was being slowly, painfully dismembered. I had little left to do but comment on the fight, but even here I was aware that Larkin was talking in Czyz's earphone from the production truck. In essence, he was calling the fight himself, using Czyz as his dummy. Well folks, Czyz was a former world champion with a lifetime in boxing, and Larkin was not. He was all show business. I wanted to hear what Czyz had to say—I felt his opinion was valuable—but, of course, I was cut out of those conversations. I wouldn't have stood for it, and I couldn't understand how Czyz could. When a network hires you for your opinion and expertise, why should you listen to a producer who has never been in boxing telling an audience what he thinks?

Unfortunately, boxing is a sport that seems easy to understand on the outside. In four weeks the average fan can be an expert, and in six weeks a network executive thinks he is master of the sport and knows as much as anyone. Well fans, he doesn't. There's more to boxing than meets the eye. It takes years of living and breathing the sport to know it. TV people will never get it. Never!

As an obvious example, Czyz has been in boxing since he was a child, but Steve Albert, the blow-by-blow man, never saw a fight in person before he came on camera, but now Albert is one of the best analysts around. When he's through with Showtime, he'll never want to see another fight, but Czyz will be a boxing man until he dies. So will I. A Jay Larkin feels he really knows all there is to know about boxing, but he doesn't. What he does know is all there is to know about televising the matches. Fourteen years of fights will do that for you.

During these changes, I had distant conversations with a warm, intelligent, gracious executive vice president named Gordon Hall, who had been with me at NBC and had treated me with much respect. I voiced my protests about the piece-by-piece demise to his friendly ear, but he could only agree with my evaluation. I had put up with greasing the skids because when the big boys decided Czyz was ready to go it alone, I'd be history.

To be fair, during this time I felt that Larkin was fighting hard to keep me. I felt he was the point of attack because that was his job. Larkin, on the other hand, had put his feet in the fire. The crown of a TV exec never sits easy. From time to time he would hint that he was having problems over me.

I knew Larkin was getting hammered from above, but I felt we could stretch the end of my career out to make it smooth, if not pleasant. Alas, that wasn't the case. He handled it badly, like a college student who gets through four years but fails the final exams. Or, if you were to see him as what he was, an actor, then I'd say he was great for the first two acts, but stunk in the final scene. He needed to polish up his people skills.

I suppose my firing did not come as a shock, although the nasty, insensitive way it took place did.

We had just finished the David Tua versus Obed Sullivan fight on June 3, 2000, at a large Vegas hotel and were headed back to the truck to watch the replays and get an idea of how it went. This fight happened to be good, and I felt our call was right on the money. Czyz had been sharp, and Steve Albert had quit addressing all comments to Czyz, so we had a clean and balanced show. I was very happy with the way the night had gone.

Larkin intercepted me outside the production truck with a big smile on his face.

"Great. Great show. Good fight, good call," he said, vigorously pumping my hand.

"I thought we had great team balance," I said in agreement. "Bobby was great tonight."

At this point the expression on his face changed, as if a Venetian blind had been pulled down, and his demeanor turned from cheerful to very heavy and dark.

"Can I speak to you for a moment?" he said, guiding me by the arm to a row of black trash cans behind the trucks.

I didn't like the feel of this. Anything that's said in an atmosphere like that couldn't be good. I stood like a criminal, waiting to hear the jury's verdict.

"This is the worst night of my life," he began, choking back tears. "I don't know how to say this." He was hemming and hawing, while I was starting to feel my guts implode.

"Try English," I told him, remembering Chris Dundee.

Larkin finally looked directly into my eyes and said, "Tonight is your last night."

I don't remember much about the conversation after that, but the enormity of this stab in the back didn't hit me until I got back to my room and was alone. No one had been told; no one knew but me. Even my wife, who usually came with me when I traveled, wasn't there to comfort me, and telling her over the phone just didn't seem right.

Actually, the bulk of my bad feelings was not the fact that I was fired. Hell, I expected that. What really bothered me was the sense of betrayal I felt from a trusted friend. I had come to Showtime to help lend credibility and acceptability to the fledgling show, and I had tied my wagon to Larkin because he seemed so honest, so down to earth, and so likeable. From the first moment I began the show, we had no contract—just a handshake from one year to the next. And somewhere along that 14-year run I had said to him, "We have a gentleman's agreement, a partners' handshake, and if they fire you, I'm gone, too." And I meant it. At the time Larkin appreciated that vow of loyalty and had responded with his own, "As long as I'm here, you're here." Those words rang in my ear all that night.

I had accepted the downswing of my career—I couldn't accept the demeaning ways the executives were chopping me to pieces. But to be told in such a cruel, insensitive way by the guy I had relied on and had supported in turn that I was finished, that was knife-twisting betrayal at its finest.

I took a plane home the next day, unable to feel anything, and met Luisita at the airport. I had a hard time not blurting out what had just been done to me, but I waited until we finally reached our parking place before I stammered, "I've got something bad to tell you."

"You've been fired. I knew it when I saw you in that fire engine red coat," she said.

She had an uncanny knack for knowing things before anyone else does. It came from her North American Indian stock.

The very loud blood-red coat had been given to me as a lark before a show once, and I had been dared to wear it, so as soon as she saw me wearing it, she knew.

We sat and talked into the night, and as usual she lifted my sagging spirit and put things into perspective.

"Listen, you have a lot of work to do yet, it may not be on television. But your life is not over. We have a gallery that needs to be run, and we have an exhibit soon. You will be off the boxing track for a while, but that doesn't mean you won't get back on. Reputation and experience have to count for something. Remember the most important thing you have is me and our love. No executive, no matter how big, can take that away. So let's go home now."

She was right, and that about sums it up. It was a good ride while it lasted.

Later Showtime invited me to write on their website and to announce my retirement on a boxing show so it would at least make them look good. But in the end, I will never forget the classless insensitivity that the Showtime executives exhibited.

I am comforted to know that fans still stop me on the street in New York, Atlanta, Miami, or anywhere I go today and say, "Hi, Doc, we miss you on HBO. You always said it like it was."

Almost famous. Oh, and Showtime was never mentioned.

✗✗✗✗✗✗✗

Looking at boxing today, there are a few areas I failed to rehabilitate that are still badly in need of reform.

I had researched blindness in older boxers and found that most of them had endured detached retinas that already had been surgically repaired. Once a retina is repaired, it can't be repaired again, so there's no way to fix it. The way I saw it, there needed to be a rule stating that a boxer should not be allowed to fight again with a surgically repaired detached retina. To me, it seemed as simple as that. It did to many other people, too. The rule was widely accepted and ready to be adopted. Blindness from boxing would be a thing of the past.

Then Sugar Ray Leonard wanted to come out of retirement to fight "Marvelous Marvin" Hagler. That shot the rule all to hell. It was Leonard—big bucks! Let him box if he wants to, the little darling.

I fought very hard. I interviewed Leonard's ophthalmologist on NBC. He was a young egomaniac, who said incredibly arrogant things when the camera was rolling.

"The eye is now stronger than before it was injured," he said.

"What? Better than when God made it?"

Here was a surgeon who actually thought he could improve on God's handiwork. What an egotistical fool!

"Actually, the surgically repaired eye is stronger than his other undamaged eye," he told me.

"Tell me, if that was your son going in that ring, would you let him fight Hagler?" I wanted to rattle him, if I could.

"I wouldn't let my son be a fighter," he said smugly, adroitly side-stepping the question.

After the interview, he came up to me almost meekly and said, "You know, I can't say this on camera, but actually, doctor to doctor, I don't believe he should fight."

I could have smashed him in the face. The nerve, the arrogance. Although he was a young man, he didn't live to see whether Leonard went blind because he died a few years after the interview. I must say, though it sounds harsh, I don't mourn his passing. Because of his egomania and arrogance, and Leonard's stubborn insistence to gamble with his eyesight, there are still plenty of blind boxers out there. There shouldn't be any.

Another losing battle of my well-intentioned cleanup campaign was to try to get boxers past their prime out of the ring before they were permanently damaged and to keep the old-timers (like Leonard) from coming back long after their bodies can handle the stress.

I was aware of the legalities involved in denying a man the right to make a living and that one has a right to chance one's destruction if one wishes. But I nonetheless dug in my heels. I wanted an arbitrary age limit of 37 to be set, if you weren't already out of the ring by then. Moreover, if you had been retired for five or more years, forget coming back. Of course, there would be exceptions, such as Archie Moore, Roberto Duran, and Muhammad Ali—all of the biggies.

All that this would mean was that the boxing commissions would have the responsibility to safeguard a boxer's health. Their first obligation would be to administering laws that primarily concerned the health and welfare of the boxer.

Most sensible commissioners agreed, and everything was ambling slowly along, coalescing into an agreement between the three boards involved. Then out of the slums of Houston, Texas, came the shambling remains of a great champion, George Foreman. He had honorably blown his winnings, maintaining a small church for 10 years. Now he was broke, and he was back. What were they to do?

I proposed the law specifically for fighters such as Foreman. It was a supreme test. Well, the boxing commission said, "This is big bucks! A legendary fight! How could we say no?" So the law folded like a Taliban tent in the night.

What they all forgot was Foreman saw Christ in a dressing room in Zaire. He got religion, founded a church, financed it, and after 10 worthwhile praiseworthy years, he found he had used up all of his savings. So, he turned to his breadwinner—prize fighting.

The restrictions on age fell by the wayside. George was over 37, hadn't fought in 10 years, and looked like the Titanic when it was sinking. He was blubbery and out of shape, to put it mildly.

I know boxing, and if I had gotten my hands on Foreman, I'd have done exactly what his promoter did. He staged a series of phony fights on TV that would net the mighty Foreman 30 knockouts and a plateful of money. However, as Foreman worked his way into shape, he began to believe he could be the champion once again. So the fights became legitimate. Foreman is a really big man with one of the heaviest punches in the history of boxing. He's tough and durable and has a very big heart. He would take a giant beating in order to land just one punch that would end the fight on the spot.

In November 1994, after countless head whippings, he found himself in the ring with a lackluster young champion by the name of Michael Moorer, who figured he'd pound Foreman to a pulp. Well, he was right about the beating, but he let Foreman hang around for too long, and as he got careless, Foreman uncorked his atom bomb punch. Down and out went Moorer, and unbelievably, Foreman was the champion once again!

I'm sure many fans said, "Hooray for George! He was right to come back."

My view is this: Foreman was right to come back for Foreman's sake, but he was very wrong for boxing's sake. In the wake of his fraudulent buildup, the barn doors opened and out tumbled every old beat-up ex-champion seeking to duplicate Foreman's feat.

Well, none did, but the beatings they sustained trying to get their championship belts back hurried them along into punch drunkenness and ultimately Parkinson's disease.

The three greatest fighters in history are Joe Louis, Sugar Ray Robinson, and Muhammad Ali. All three have one thing in common: Filled with self-delusion, all three fought years past their prime and all three suffered incapacitating illnesses. Tough old Foreman broke that record, though, and made it easy for fighters to punch their way into the neurological ward. Even Duran retired at 50. Disgraceful.

Why Foreman hasn't shown signs of punch drunkenness is a mystery to me. He changed his character for the better and now is a very pleasant, agreeable man who charms TV audiences and has opened up many avenues to amass a fortune. I hope he has hung up the gloves for good.

I always refused to work a Foreman fight, and you can imagine how the tight-ass execs felt about that. With NBC, I had an open mike to blast Foreman every chance I got, but Showtime had trouble swallowing my refusal to call Foreman's phony fights. I won, but they weren't happy.

✗✗✗✗✗✗

I felt the same way about women's boxing as I did about Foreman. For years, I had watched as masculine he-she's came to the Fifth Street Gym to try to fight professionally, but thankfully, Chris Dundee ran them off. Then I personally blocked their appearance on NBC. I didn't want boxing to turn into a freak show, and I was convinced women would damage their health, and, besides, I naïvely thought, what red-blooded male would want to see two females flailing at one another?

When I was at Showtime and not in an executive position, they caved in to King's demand that they put female boxers on the undercard. I fought like hell to prevent it, but I lost. However, I would never call a woman's bout—and never have.

All of my medical training directed to avoid physical blows to the breasts of women. The prevailing thought was that one good blow to the breast could damage sensitive tissue that would develop into breast cancer in time. Breast cancer in a middle-aged woman is no day in the park. It is a very serious matter to be avoided at all cost.

Now come a few masculine women willing to overlook medical warnings and to risk cancer in middle age by having their breasts punched repeatedly in a fight. Remember, also, that these women train every day and are punched every day. Some women even work out with men, although why that outrage is allowed is beyond me.

The effect of hard physical training and physical abuse also contributes to menstrual irregularities and hormonal changes. Granted, not many of the women I saw fighting were worrying about having children and raising a family, but still, that feminine function is seriously affected.

Can we make a woman protect herself from cancer or from physical and physiological damage? We stopped smoking all over the place, why not boxing? Why shouldn't we protect women from even the possibility of cancer of the breast?

Besides the obvious objections I had as a doctor, I had more serious reservations about women in boxing. They had no ruling body, no specific rules for women and no one to check records. Once, on Showtime, we had a black model who drove all night from Atlanta to get on a TV fight with us. Result? Knockout in one round. The truth was she had never had one professional fight. It was disgraceful.

For every Christy Martin, there are 100 girls who can't fight a lick. I personally love Martin, the "Coal Miner's Daughter," as a person. She showed up bright as hell—she was a teacher—happily married to her coach. She dressed in pink and was pretty as a picture, and she could fight! The problem was they couldn't find any gal in the United States or Europe who came close to her skills. Martin swept through 30 mismatches. She was a big hit for King, who put her on every Showtime bout. The matches were so easy I couldn't even watch them. And I'm very sorry to say, I saw beautiful Martin change into a boxing pug.

When she was starting out, I was friendly with Martin and her husband. As I was warning her to get out as soon as possible, she said to me, "Don't worry. As soon as we make $30,000 to put a down payment on our house, we're out of here."

"No, you won't be," I said sadly and told her Leonard had said a similar thing to me—that as soon as he got $1 million in the bank he would be gone. I told him he wouldn't, too, and he stayed on until they almost carried his one-eyed self out of the ring.

Now Martin's once beautiful nose is thick and bulbous. Her eyebrows have scars and are getting heavy. Her beautiful innocent face is now gone, and a gargoyle is forming up. What a shame. I guess she has made over $1 million, and I hope she is happy with what she has accomplished, beating up dozens of untalented, unprofessional girls who stepped into the ring hoping to become the next Christy Martin. And, if you need to ask, Martin is still boxing.

Occasionally, a new vice president would come take a shot at me about women's boxing. Once, Larkin, the vice president in charge of Showtime boxing, who was at that time my best friend, took a weak shot at my position.

"I checked with my wife's gynecologist, and he says he can't see why you connect punches on the breast to breast cancer."

Well, Larkin was no intellectual giant. As calmly as I could, I pointed out to him that he and his gynecologist were at least 12 inches south of what we are examining. A gynecologist has no more business in breast carcinoma than a urologist. And an actor—as Larkin had been—has no business at all discussing it with a legitimate authority. Case closed.

They came in waves, those empty-headed executives, or they sent the producer, David Dinkins, but all met the same fate. I worked 25 years broadcasting boxing and never did a women's boxing event.

Still, during my career in boxing, we made great progress in protecting the fighters and diminishing the number of deaths in the ring. Maybe one day someone will see the light on old boxers and women in the ring.

XXXXXXX

Ever since Showtime unceremoniously dumped me, I have found myself as busy as ever. You can find me nearly every day at my home in the Miami area, writing a novel or nonfiction, or painting. I will continue to paint every day until I die. I love it.

I've had offers to return to television to do boxing. There are projects for children's charities and other work. I listen to them all and do what I can.

In my private life I was blessed by an exceptional human being, my wife, Luisita, who presented me with a reason to live, and a perfect daughter, Tina. They have made everything easy and fun. If I had to sum up my life, it simply this: Never Quit! Never Quit! Never!

XXXXXXX

Now I'm standing at the end of the road, looking back at a hectic, fun-filled life and ruminating. Was this what J.B., my dad, had in mind for me? Did I live up to his code of conduct? Would he have been proud of me?

I am happy that he gave me a road map of life. I tried to follow his opinions and his rules of conduct.

"Be a man," he said, "Stand up to your beliefs, don't back down, don't quit."

I think I did that.

"Maximize your talents, don't be afraid to take chances to follow new paths."

I certainly did that.

"Use your education and background to help the poor. Alleviate pain, hunger, and disease. Always see how to use your position (doctor, writer, painter), to help others along in life."

"Do the right thing. Be a good person. Love everyone as you would like to be loved."

All of this, I think I've done. I am looking forward one day to seeing Pop and Grandfather again and getting a pat on the back.